Dogs, Diet, and Disease

An Owner's Guide to Diabetes Mellitus, Pancreatitis, Cushing's Disease & More

Caroline D. Levin RN

Foreword by Albert J. Simpson DVM

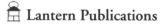 Lantern Publications

Illustrations and photographs by Caroline Levin (except where otherwise noted).

Cover photographs: (Top) Pat Stevens and "Ginger," (Center) Natalie Shellans and "Bouncer," (Bottom) Joeanne Butler and "Liza."

Second Printing, June, 2001
Printed in Canada

 Lantern Publications
    18709 S. Grasle Road
    Oregon City, OR 97045

ISBN 0-9672253-2-9
LCCN 2001116527

❯•❮

Dedication

This book is dedicated to the memory of my beloved Beeren. He was a real dog's dog, a joyful, ready-to-play, come-when-called kind of dog. He was taken far too soon.

Losing him drove me to learn all I could about canine disease and wellness. If this knowledge can help another, then Beeren's passing was not in vain.

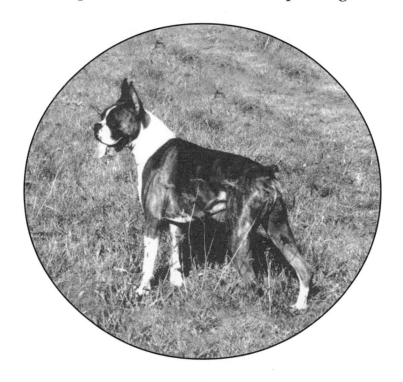

Dornlea's Spirit Moves Me CDX
June 12, 1993 — December 15, 2000

"Dogs lives are too short; it's their only fault, really."
— Alice Sligh Turnbull

Acknowledgements

I would like to extend my sincere thanks to Dr. Albert James Simpson, a wonderful veterinarian and teacher. His time and knowledge have been greatly appreciated.

Many thanks to the canine nutritionists who have shared their expertise with me: Jennifer Boniface, MS; Lisa Newman, PhD; and especially Lew Olsen, PhD. Their willingness to teach helped make this book a reality.

Thanks, too, to the dog owners who have repeatedly spoken with me about their dogs and their experiences: Jodie Jeweler, Kerry Meydem, Linda Glass, Karen Flocker, Shari Burghart, Judy Simmons, Yvonne Mantell, Kathy Partridge, Donna Bartkow, Leslie Lawson, Susan Flewelling, Judy Dick, Walter Orzechowski, Pam Hunt, Lori Zech, and Jean Sweezie.

I am grateful to Pam Lardear for sharing pictures of her dog "Kate," and to Pat and Joel Stevens and their Labrador, "Ginger," for graciously posing for photographs. Thanks also to my mother, Natalie Shellans, for posing with "Bouncer," English Mastiff; to my brother, Timothy Shellans, for posing with "Columbo," English Mastiff; and to Joeanne Butler for posing with "Liza," Miniature Schnauzer.

I am deeply grateful to Tamara Coli for raising beautiful puppies on real food, and for her insight, and comments on this subject.

I would also like to acknowledge the contributions of the many other dog owners who have answered my questions over the years — too many to name, but all of them important. I hope that when they recognize their comments herein, they realize my gratitude.

I thank my family and friends, who continually support me as I plow through these projects. This one was especially challenging. As always, I am grateful to my husband, Daniel, without whom my books would not be possible, and to my editor, Patty Bonnstetter, for all her hard work. Finally, I offer my gratitude to Deborah Wood, fellow dog writer and trainer, who kept me going when I was ready to call it quits.

Contents

Preface ix
About the Author xi
Foreword xiii

Chapter 1
Dealing With Loss.. 1
Denial 2
Anger 2
Bargaining 3
Depression 3
Acceptance 3
Children and Loss 5

Chapter 2
The Doctor-Client Relationship 7
The Veterinarian's Part 7
The Dog Owner's Part 8
Treatment Philosophies 8

Chapter 3
Normal Canine Metabolism and Endocrine Function 11
Normal Canine Anatomy 11
Normal Canine Metabolism 13

Chapter 4
Diabetes Mellitus.. 17
Abnormal Canine Metabolism — Diabetes 17
Types of Diabetes 19
Causes of Diabetes 19
Autoimmune Disease 20
Prevalence 21
Diagnosing Diabetes Mellitus... 21

Chapter 5
Cushing's Disease and Excess Cortisol Production 23
Abnormal Canine Metabolism — Cushing's Disease 23
Types of Hyperadrenocorticism 26
Causes of Hyperadrenocorticism 27
Prevalence 27
Diagnosing Cushing's Disease 27

Chapter 6
Pancreatic Disease 33
Abnormal Canine Metabolism – Pancreatic Disease 33
Types of Pancreatitis 35
Other Pancreatic Diseases 36
Causes of Pancreatitis 36
Prevalence 37
Diagnosing Pancreatic Disease 37

Chapter 7
What Causes These Diseases? 39
Commercial Diets 39
The Benefits of Feeding Commercial Pet Foods 40
The Drawbacks of Feeding Commercial Pet Foods 40
Protein Sources in Commercial Foods 42
Enzymes 42
Altered Amino Acids 44
Slowed Digestion 44
Bioavailability 45
Fiber in Commercial Foods 45
Chemicals in Commercial Foods 46
Grains and the Endocrine Pancreas 46
A Review of the Immune System 47
Fats in Commercial Foods 51
Summary 52

Chapter 8
Dietary Management 55
A Review of Commercial Diets 55
More Wholesome Options for Feeding 56
Diets Prepared at Home 57
Preparing a Home-cooked Diet 57
The Benefits of Feeding Home-cooked Diets 61
The Drawbacks of Feeding Home-cooked Diets 61
Raw Food Diets 62
Preparing a Raw Food Diet 64
The Benefits of Feeding Raw Food Diets 65

The Drawbacks of Feeding Raw Food Diets 66
Variations in Homemade Diets 66
Switching Diets 66
Snacks, Treats, and How to Hide Medications 67
Water Consumption 69
Changes in Body Weight 70
Other Oral Aids 70

Chapter 9
Caring for Dogs With Diabetes Mellitus.. 73
An Overview of Insulin Activity 73
Types of Insulin 74
Timing meals with injections 77
Insulin Bottles and Label Information 80
Syringes and Needles 81
Reusing Needles and Syringes 82
Syringe Disposal 83
Insulin Storage and Handling 83
Preparing Injections 84
Pre-filling Syringes and Enlisting the Help of Others 87
Giving Insulin Injections 88
Injections Gone Wrong / Complications 96
Hypoglycemic Incidents 98
Regulating Glucose Levels 100
Blood Glucose Testing at the Veterinary Clinic 101
Subjectively Monitoring Clinical Signs 102
Urine Glucose Testing 103
Home Blood Glucose Testing 105
Difficulties in Getting Regulated 115
Exercise and the Diabetic Dog 120
Traveling With a Diabetic Dog 121
Traveling Without Your Dog 121

Chapter 10
Caring for Dogs With Cushing's Disease and Excess Cortisol 123
Surgical Treatment 123
Medical Treatment 123
Comfort Measures 127

Chapter 11
Caring for Dogs With Pancreatic Disease 131
Treating Acute Pancreatitis 131
Treating Chronic Pancreatitis 132
Treating Pancreatic Enzyme Insufficiency (PEI) 133

Chapter 12
Additional Health Concerns **135**
Physical Assessment 135
Infections 136
Renal (Kidney) Problems 140
Treating Incontinence 140
Thyroid Disease 144
Calcinosis Cutis 145
Ophthalmic Issues 145
Surgical Considerations 154

Closing 155

Suppliers 159

Glossary 165

Bibliography 171

Index 173

Preface

I was caught off guard the first few times dog owners asked me questions about managing canine diabetes. As with the subject of canine blindness, it became apparent that there was a need for educational material on this topic, as well. So began the year-and-half-long effort to write this book.

Halfway through the project, my gorgeous, six-year-old Boxer, Beeren, fell ill and died in just a matter of days. While his most significant sign was respiratory distress (fluid in his lungs), he was actually diagnosed with IgA deficiency. It came as quite a surprise.

After recovering from this loss, I continued my work. I noticed that my diabetes research also began to answer questions I had about IgA deficiency and autoimmune disease. Not only did I understand why I had lost my *six*-year-old Boxer, but I also learned about the inflammatory bowel disease, chronic skin infections, incontinence and cancer that had taken my *seven*-year-old Boxer, Liebschen, shortly before.

Dog owners sent me encouragement as I continued writing. They also sent me queries. They asked me to include information about Cushing's disease, pancreatitis, and dietary issues, too. I soon realized that these problems were closely related. My little diabetes book evolved into a dissertation on immune disorders, metabolic disease, digestive problems, and canine nutrition.

You will learn many helpful things from this book. Some might make you slap your forehead and cry, "Of course! Those are exactly the symptoms my dog has!" Others things may surprise you greatly, so much so, that you may not want to believe them. With this book, you can help your present dog have a better quality of life and spare your future pets a lifetime of chronic disease. Share what you learn with your breeder, your veterinarians, and friends.

In the dog fancy, male dogs are usually referred to as exactly that, "dogs," while females are referred to as "bitches." For ease in writing this book, I've chosen to refer to all canines, both male and female as "dogs" or "he." This does not represent a higher incidence of illness among males. (I have also referred to all owners as "he.") ✳

X

About the Author

With a unique combination of personal and professional experiences, Caroline Levin has created an important resource book for dog owners. "Dogs, Diet, and Disease" examines some of the most serious digestive, metabolic, and autoimmune diseases diagnosed in dogs today.

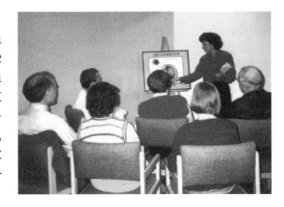

Levin's experience in healthcare began as an ophthalmic registered nurse. After a decade of nursing, Levin left this field to manage an ophthalmic veterinary clinic. It was here that she realized the desperate need blind-dog owners had for educational material. Since then, she has written the first two works on this topic: "Living With Blind Dogs" and "Blind Dog Stories."

Periodically, Levin's readers contacted her with questions about canine diabetes. She realized that there was a need for educational material on this topic, too. Simultaneously, Levin lost her show-ring obedience dog to an autoimmune disease. These events compelled her to search for answers. She scrutinized the current literature and talked with dozens of dog owners, diabetes educators, and canine nutritionists. Levin drew on her own nursing background, as well. The result is this, Levin's third, and perhaps most important, book.

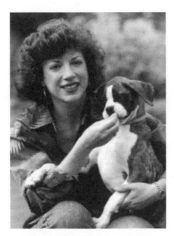

Photo courtesy of Vern Witake

Caroline Levin is also an award-winning dog trainer. She has an in-depth understanding of canine behavior and the methods used to successfully train dogs. She shows her dogs in AKC obedience trials and the new sport of musical canine freestyle. Levin is frequently requested as a guest speaker and has written for a variety of publications. ✳

Foreword

"We thought she was just drinking too much water, we had no idea that dogs could get diabetes. Do we have to put her to sleep? Do we have to give her insulin shots? How did this happen? We give her the best care possible."

After being in the practice of veterinary medicine for more than 20 years, I have seen the tears, the confusion, even guilt, when owners learn that their dog has diabetes. Informing a pet owner that his or her dog has diabetes mellitus is not an easy job. They ask questions regarding cause, effect, and management of this disease. In those first few emotional minutes in the exam room, the pet owner is overwhelmed with information. Most of it makes sense at the time, but a few days or weeks later, many of the same questions recur. Consequently, many dogs are put to sleep (euthanized) either in the early stages of trying to manage the disease, or sometimes without making any management attempt at all.

This book provides reassuring answers to these questions in an easy-to-read format, an owner's manual for the conscientious and caring pet owner. Caroline Levin has accomplished the task of putting a holistic approach to the management of diabetes mellitus. She has looked at the other organs, especially the adrenal gland, for their roles in stress and its relationship to the immune system. She includes the role of dietary factors as both a major contributing cause and as an effective management strategy for the diabetic condition. Related conditions are covered in chapters explaining hormonal dysfunction such as Cushing's disease.

Ms. Levin's book is a wealth of practical ideas on what and how to feed dogs with diabetes, as well as sound advice on traditional treatments, including insulin injections and exercise. This book should be recommended to all those individuals caring for a diabetic dog, and is a "must read" for their veterinarians.

Albert J. Simpson DVM

Chapter 1

Dealing With Loss

Many people feel overwhelmed when their dog is diagnosed with a chronic illness. Some may feel overwhelmed after simply skimming through the pages of this book. Others may cry or feel anger. All of these are normal and natural reactions. As one dog owner explains it, "There is a particular type of grief we experience when someone we love goes from being 'whole' to being 'handicapped.'"

Some owners are sad for their dog's sake, wondering what quality of life they can expect for their dog. Others are sad for their own sake. They may ask themselves questions such as:

"Will I still love my dog as much as I did before the disease?"
"Will he be as good as everyone else's dog?"
"Will my friends and family pity my dog?"
"Will I be able to provide the necessary care?"
"Will my dog have a happy life or will he be miserable?"

Author Elisabeth Kubler-Ross is well known for her work in the area of grief management. She has outlined five stages people typically experience as they cope with loss: denial, anger, bargaining, depression, and finally, acceptance. This progression can certainly be applied to the dog owner as he adjusts to his dog's new condition.

Grieving is like a roller-coaster ride, with many ups and downs. People experience these stages in varying sequences. Some move through one stage, only to return to it at a later time. Other people may even employ more than one coping mechanism at a time.

The way in which an individual copes may depend on the nature of the relationship he has with the dog. Someone closely bonded may naturally experience a tremendous grief experience. Other recent losses in a person's life can compound the grief as well.

Denial

Initially, a common way to cope with loss is through denial. Denial protects the mind from the bad news being received. A dog owner may seek out a second or third medical opinion, in hopes of hearing that the disease was misdiagnosed or that the dog will experience a miraculous recovery.

When a dog owner is in denial, the situation may seem unreal to him. He may continue daily activities just as if the dog were not ill, even to the point of withholding medical care. During this phase, an owner may distance himself emotionally from his pet. By reducing contact with the dog, the owner can avoid facing his own pain.

Anger

Eventually, denial gives way to a stage of anger. This is a time when a dog owner may say to himself, "This is so unfair. Why did this happen to my dog!?"

In normal instances, humans are the caretakers, guardians, and rule-makers for their dogs. In the face of sudden illness, a dog owner may feel that he is no longer in control of the situation. This may contribute to his level of anger. An inability to ensure a pet's well being can be enormously frustrating.

It is not uncommon for the dog owner to have angry feelings toward the veterinary staff as well. In the dog-owner's mind, not only did the veterinarian make this diagnosis, but neither is he able to cure the problem!

Anger may also be expressed toward friends and family members, frequently taking the form of criticism. It is important to recognize that such outbursts may only be expressions of the dog-owner's grief.

It is even possible for the dog owner to express anger toward the dog. He doesn't truly blame the dog for somehow "catching" an illness. He is simply frustrated and wishes he could restore the dog's previous level of health. Happily, our dogs are immensely forgiving creatures and may never remember this stage.

Guilt feelings can be associated with the anger stage. The owner may question his own care of the dog and wonder if something he did could have caused his dog's disease. Such guilt may manifest itself in a number of unhealthy ways. Excessive coddling of the dog is one example.

Bargaining

The anger stage sometimes gives way to a bargaining stage. An owner may believe at some level that if denial and anger did not resolve this problem, he may be able to make a deal or bargain for a cure.

The bargaining is usually done secretly, with a "Higher Power." One example might be, "If you make my dog well, I will never raise my voice to her again!" Bargaining is a way to keep hope alive. This phase is often short-lived and the dog owner may progress to a state of depression.

Depression

Depression or sorrow may set in when the signs of illness can no longer be denied. Some owners mistakenly believe that chronic disease will be a death sentence or, at least, a major disability for their dog. They mistakenly believe that their most enjoyable activities — such as hiking in the woods or running together on the beach — will be lost.

While friends might try to cheer the grieving pet owner, it is important to allow the transition through this stage. It is important for each dog owner to give himself permission to grieve. Sorrow is actually a healing emotion. It allows an individual to prepare for the future and accept the realities of caring for his dog.

The time it takes for a person to move through this stage can vary greatly. There is no predetermined timetable. Eventually the feelings of sadness and helplessness will give way to feelings of acceptance, the final stage.

Acceptance

Acceptance is reached when an individual has had time to work through all the previous stages. There is no average time for this process. As one dog owner put it, "It takes as long as it takes." Talking with sympathetic friends and enjoying the smallest of pleasures with your dog may help.

Once a dog owner is no longer isolated or in denial, no longer angry or depressed, he reaches a stage of resolution. Now he becomes less of a patient himself and more of a caregiver to his dog. It is at this point that healthcare information is best received.

If an owner has not really reached the acceptance stage, he may have negative reactions to caring for his dog. He may have difficulty remembering details about treatment. This is an important concept for both veterinary staff and the owners of newly diagnosed dogs.

As the acceptance stage is reached, it is valuable to consider this question: What are the "jobs" dogs do in this day and age?

With the exception of a few dogs that truly earn their keep as herding dogs, hunting dogs, or service dogs, most dogs today are generally unemployed. Our dogs have only a few basic functions in our homes: they alert us to visitors at the door, they want to cuddle in one form or another, and they make us laugh. **Dogs suffering from digestive/metabolic diseases can do all these things as well as other dogs.**

While illness will certainly have an effect on your dog, it is important to remember that current treatments are highly effective. This is confirmed by the number of dogs successfully living today with diabetes, Cushing's disease, and pancreatitis. Appropriate treatment will significantly reduce the symptoms of these diseases, extend a dog's life span, and maintain the normal activities of daily living and recreation.

This book will give you the information and confidence to help you and your dog return to a sense of being "whole." You will regain a sense of control over your dog's healthcare. With time, patience, and commitment, living with a canine illness will simply become part of your daily routine.

It is easy to think that you must be an instant expert — that you must know so many things at once. Learning about healthcare is more like a journey. Each day you will understand more about the disease and how your dog reacts. Turn to sections in the book that are most pressing to you now, and read other sections as your schedule permits. Dealing with one thing at a time will help keep it all manageable.

As you progress with training and your dog with treatment, you may find yourselves bonding more closely. Besides providing your dog with life-saving treatment, pet care tends to deepen trust and improve communication. There is a special relationship that develops when you care for a dog with special needs.

Some owners explain that they do have to juggle their schedules a bit to care for their dogs, but the fact that they *depend* on a schedule brings them closer together. Giving insulin injections and other medications becomes a bonding experience. Many owners provide a special play session right afterward to remind their dogs that they are still normal in the important ways. They spend extra time together *because* of the dog's condition.

It is also valuable, however, to keep balance in your life. Since these illnesses are long-term conditions, it is important for the caregiver to avoid burnout. If your schedule demands that you miss one of your dog's injections, pills, drops, or if you just need a break from your day-to-day responsibilities, it may be possible to have a trusted friend or family member step in. If the dog must miss a single insulin injection, or dose of medication, once in while, it will probably not adversely affect him in the long run.

Children and Loss

Try to include children in the grieving process. Children often share a very strong bond to the family pet. They may experience feelings of anger and worry. Including children in these painful times teaches them several things: that is good to express emotion and fear, and how to develop coping skills. As with yourself, give children permission to grieve.

Children can obviously sense when something is wrong. Avoiding the issue or lying about the dog's condition could result in lack of trust or irrational fear on the child's part. Adults who show respect for children's feelings help them build confidence in dealing with loss.

Openness and honesty encourage questions from the child. Straightforward answers are the best tactic. Be patient, as children may need to repeatedly revisit issues. Try to include all family members in the process of education and pet care, whenever appropriate. ✳

Chapter 2

The Doctor-Client Relationship

Optimum canine healthcare requires a trusting relationship between dog owner and veterinarian. Both parties must be active participants in the dog's care. Both must communicate effectively.

Several things contribute to the success of this relationship. These include the dog owner's learning style, his level of motivation, and the veterinarian's teaching style and experience. It is also of prime importance that the dog owner and doctor have shared philosophies about general pet care and feeding issues.

The Veterinarian's Part

Some dog owners seek out the care of specialists, veterinarians who specialize in the field of internal medicine and the management of diseases such as diabetes, pancreatitis and Cushing's disease. Other owners have good experiences with their general-practice, hometown veterinarians. In these cases, the doctors do aggressive research to educate themselves and their clients. They are willing to consult with specialists or more experienced veterinarians.

Still other dog owners have poor results in this situation. They believe that doctors who are inexperienced in treating their dog's disease are not current on the best therapies. Some owners become anxious that their dog's care is not as progressive as it might be. Since each dog will react differently to treatment, a doctor's level of experience can be a valuable asset.

To help decide this issue, many dog owners find it helpful to ask a few interview-type questions of the doctor. They want to know how many other patients the doctor has had, or is treating, with a specific condition. And they want to know how these pets have generally fared.

The veterinarian's practice style is another important element in a successful relationship. Some veterinarians may not be accustomed to including their clients as partners in the delivery of canine healthcare. Others are more forthcoming with their findings and opinions. They include the pet owner in discussions and decision-making.

Some brilliant clinicians, when faced with a hectic schedule, may appear brusque to clients. Most pet owners value bedside manner as much as technical competence. They want to feel comfortable asking questions of the doctor.

Finally, some doctors are simply better teachers than are others. If a doctor does not explain things in a way that is understandable to each particular dog owner, it will not be helpful to the dog.

The Dog Owner's Part

Even the best veterinarian, however, cannot deliver effective care without the active participation of the dog owner. The owner must be willing to learn about the disease and ask for clarification. He must accept his role as a caregiver. And he must learn to assess the dog's condition, communicate this to the doctor, and make informed decisions.

In addition, it is important that the veterinarian and dog owner have a shared philosophy about basic dog care. Since treatment plans can include diet, exercise, medications, supplements, and blood tests, it is important to have a doctor who will support your educated decisions and whatever strong beliefs you may have.

When there are glaring differences in these matters, it can be beneficial to seek a second opinion. (This is a very different scenario than the case of the dog owner in denial, searching for a miraculous cure.) Getting a second opinion is common in healthcare and most doctors are not insulted by it. Dog owners sometimes ask their friends for recommendations, or consult the telephone directory, veterinary teaching hospital, or state veterinary association for a specialist.

A second opinion should also be sought when your veterinarian expresses hesitancy in treating your dog's disease or perfunctorily instructs you to euthanize an otherwise healthy pet. A trusting, open relationship is vital to the successful treatment of your dog. He is a silent participant in all of this and you are his advocate.

Treatment Philosophies

There are two general approaches to caring for chronically ill dogs. In the first approach, veterinarians realize that caring for such pets can be a strain on families and can result in a sense of burnout. These doctors are concerned with keeping care simple and manageable for dog owners.

The second approach is a more aggressive one. It is usually pursued by people who want to do everything they can to maximize their dog's health. These are people who embrace the role of the caregiver and try to learn all they can about the disease.

Neither approach is wrong. Just as all dogs are different, so are their owners. People face many commitments in their lives, professional, personal, family, and financial. What works in one family may not be a realistic option for another family. This book is written with both of these approaches in mind. It will offer a variety of options for you to consider and discuss with your veterinarian.

Also important to remember is that every dog responds to treatment differently. While various standards do exist for such things as medication dosages, calorie levels, etc., individual dogs often respond outside these parameters. A good treatment plan will be flexible. It will take into account details that are particular to you and your dog. ✻

Chapter 3

Normal Canine Metabolism and Endocrine Function

To discuss the variety of illnesses that plague dogs today, we must first examine normal canine anatomy, metabolism, and immune-system function. These processes are intricately linked to one another. The following brief descriptions are not intended to be comprehensive, but rather prepare the reader for discussions yet to come.

Normal Canine Anatomy

The **stomach** is the organ in which digestion actually begins for the dog, since dogs do not chew their food, but gulp it, instead. Unlike some other species, dogs do not have many of the molars needed to grind and mechanically break down food.

The **small intestine** is the portion of the gastrointestinal (GI) tract that follows the stomach. It is here that the majority of digestion occurs, including chemical breakdown and absorption of nutrients.

The **pancreas** is a glandular organ located in the abdomen, just posterior to the stomach. It empties into the small intestine and is considered to be both a digestive organ and an endocrine gland. Accordingly, it has two distinct functions. One portion

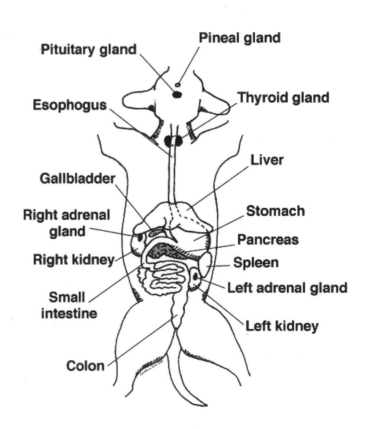

Pituitary gland
Pineal gland
Esophogus
Thyroid gland
Gallbladder
Liver
Right adrenal gland
Stomach
Right kidney
Pancreas
Spleen
Small intestine
Left adrenal gland
Left kidney
Colon

of the pancreas produces insulin. This portion is referred to as the **endocrine pancreas**. The other portion of the gland is called the **exocrine pancreas**. That portion produces digestive enzymes that help chemically break down food into useable nutrients.

The names of most enzymes end in the suffix "–ase." For example, **protease** digests proteins, **amylase** digests carbohydrates, and **lipase** digests fats (lipids). Digestive enzymes are secreted in a water-based solution. This solution flows into the small intestine via the pancreatic duct.

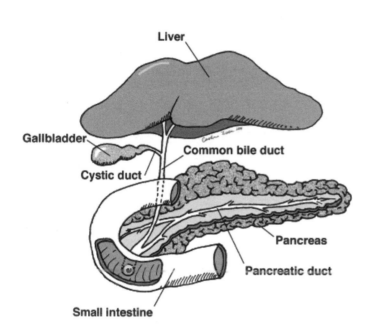

The **liver** is located alongside the stomach. It performs a multitude of jobs. It produces bile — a salty, yellowish fluid that plays an important part in the digestion of dietary fats. The liver is also the body's cleansing organ, modifying and detoxifying active substances in the bloodstream. These include hormones, medications, and waste products such as bilirubin, a yellow pigment.

The **gallbladder** is situated alongside the liver. It functions as a storage tank for bile. When food enters the small intestine, the gallbladder secretes bile to help digest dietary lipids. En route to the small intestine, bile mixes with enzymes in the common bile duct.

The **large intestine** is also referred to as the **colon**. It moves digested matter toward the rectum. One of its main functions is to reabsorb water from the GI tract, including the water that is secreted with digestive enzymes.

The **kidneys** adjust the chemical composition of the blood as necessary. The kidneys also filter the blood of poisons, body wastes, and impurities. These impurities collect and concentrate in the dog's urine. They are excreted from the body when the dog urinates.

Located near the kidneys are two small endocrine glands known as the **adrenal glands**. These glands produce a number of natural hormone/steroids, including **cortisol**. Cortisol is a beneficial and crucial chemical in the healthy dog. It orchestrates a vast number of biological tasks in the body including metabolism and the immune-system response. In normal cases, the adrenal glands secrete cortisol only as it is needed.

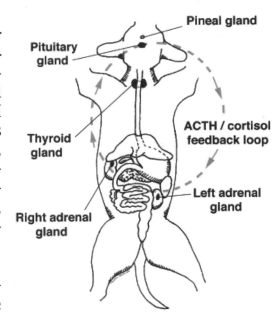

Cortisol secretion is controlled by another hormone called **adrenocorticotrophic hormone,** (also known as **ACTH.**) ACTH is produced in the **pituitary**, an endocrine gland located at the base of the brain. When ACTH is released into the bloodstream, it stimulates the adrenal glands to release cortisol. Later, when the pituitary gland recognizes that sufficient levels of cortisol are present, the pituitary gland curtails the release of ACTH, which, in turn. halts the production of cortisol. This is known as a feedback loop.

Thyroid hormone is produced in the butterfly-shaped **thyroid gland** located in the neck. This hormone regulates the body's metabolic rate. Nestled behind the thyroid gland are the **parathyroid glands.** They produce **parathyroid hormone** which controls calcium metabolism.

The **lymphatic system** is a network of tiny vessels that are similar to, but separate from, blood vessels. The lymphatic system produces many of the white blood cells needed to mount an immune response in the body.

An intimate relationship exists between the immune system, hormone production, and dietary vitamins and minerals. **Calcium** is required for dental and skeletal bone strength. Calcium also plays a role in muscle contraction and glandular secretions. **Phosphorus** is found in many types of cell membranes and maintains the pH balance of the body. **Magnesium** is necessary for a vast number of biochemical processes including metabolism, energy production, muscle relaxation and nervous system function. Magnesium activates more than 75% of metabolic enzymes in the body. It controls the enzymes in cell membranes that maintain sodium and potassium balance. This relationship is essential to water balance in the body.

Vitamin E and **Vitamin A** are necessary for normal vision and peripheral nervous system function. In humans, sufficient amounts of vitamin E are normally stored in the pituitary and adrenal glands. **Vitamin C** and the **B vitamins** play important roles in supporting immune system function. **Vitamin D** assists the pancreas to produce insulin and helps the immune system differentiate between friend and foe. It also orchestrates the process of calcium absorption: Vitamin D enters the body in an inactive state. Processes in the kidneys and liver activate it. Once activated, it is called vitamin D hormone. Vitamin D hormone regulates serum levels of calcium by pulling it from the diet or from skeletal bone. The kidney's production rate of Vitamin D, in turn, is regulated by parathyroid hormone.

Normal Canine Metabolism

Every cell in the canine body requires a source of energy to live and work. Dogs eat a variety of fats, carbohydrates, and proteins to satisfy this need. Unlike the case in humans, the digestive process in dogs does not begin until food reaches the stomach. Here, strong hydrochloric acids begin to break apart the food. The stomach also secretes the enzyme protease, which begins the process of breaking down protein.

As food passes from the stomach into the small intestine, it stimulates the pancreas to release amylase, lipase, and more protease. Up to this point, these enzymes have been inactive and stored in the pancreas. It is crucial that they remain inactive during storage, since they might otherwise digest the pancreas itself (**auto-digestion**).

Digestive enzymes are released through the pancreatic duct to the small intestine. The pancreas also secretes an alkaline solution at this time. This solution provides the chemical environment necessary to activate the enzymes. Bile is simultaneously secreted by the gall bladder to aid in the digestion of lipids.

Carbohydrates

Amylase separates carbohydrates into smaller and smaller fragments with the result being **glucose**, a simple sugar molecule. It is the primary nutrient used by the brain and nervous system.

Glucose is transported from the digestive tract to the various cells in the body via the blood stream. The level of glucose in the bloodstream is referred to as **blood glucose** or **blood sugar**. Once the glucose molecules reach their destination, they must cross cell membranes to enter and nourish the cells. This crossing is accomplished with the help of **insulin,** a hormone produced by specialized **beta cells** (also known as **Islet cells**) in the endocrine pancreas.

In normal dogs, the presence of glucose in the bloodstream stimulates the beta cells to produce a corresponding amount of insulin which is then released into the bloodstream. When insulin molecules reach the various cells of the body, they attach to special areas on the cell walls known as receptors.

To illustrate this activity, imagine a hotel doorman holding open the door for his guests. Think of the hotel as the cell and the guest as the glucose. The doorman would play the role of insulin and the doorknob would be the receptor. The doorman allows the guests into the hotel much as **insulin allows passage of glucose into the cell.**

The body maintains several protective, backup systems to ensure that the cells are always fed. In the first system, the dog's body stores excess glucose for use at a later time. For example, just after mealtime, there is a great excess of glucose available — much more than the dog immediately needs. With the help of insulin, the body stores this excess glucose in the liver and various large muscles. This stored form of glucose is known as **glycogen**. When the cells become hungry, between meals and during sleep, the body can access the glycogen. The body secretes the hormone glucogon, which releases glycogen from storage banks in the liver.

The body can even create glucose from its own sources when food is not available. In cases of prolonged hunger, the body secretes a third hormone, **cortisol**, which tells the body to convert muscle protein (**catabolism**) or body fat (**lipolysis**) into glucose. In normal cases, these intricate systems maintain the blood glucose (bg) level at a range between 80 mg/dl and 120 mg/dl.

In the United States, blood glucose levels are measured in milligrams per deciliter (mg/dl). Elsewhere in the world, blood glucose levels are measured in millimoles per liter (mmol/l). To convert the figures discussed in this text (mg/dl) to mmol/l, divide by a factor of 18.2. To check your math, remember that 10 mmol/l = 180.2 mg/dl.

Proteins

In the dog, protein is broken down by a double dose of digestive enzymes. The stomach secretes pepsin and the pancreas secretes protease. If the system is working well, protein is broken down into very small chains of **amino acids**, the building blocks of all protein. To illustrate this concept, imagine a pearl necklace. The necklace itself is a dietary protein. Each individual pearl is an amino acid. To nourish the body, the necklace must be separated into small strands consisting of only a few pearls each.

Proteins are the primary nutrients used to build and repair muscle tissue in the body. They contribute to a host of normal body functions. Almost half of the amino acids required for life and wellness must be supplied by the diet. These are called essential amino acids. (The remaining amino acids are manufactured by the body.) As with glucose, the bloodstream transports protein fragments from the digestive tract to the various cells of the body.

Fats (Lipids)

Just as carbohydrates are broken down into simple sugars, and proteins are broken down into amino acids, dietary fats (or "lipids" to the nutritionist) are broken down into **fatty acids**. The digestion of dietary fats, however, is a little more involved than the digestion of other nutrients. This is because digestive enzymes are delivered to the small intestine in a solution of water. Since oil (fats) and water don't mix, the enzymes have difficulty attaching to the lipid molecules. If they can not attach, they can not break the molecular bonds.

To solve this problem, **bile** is secreted by the gallbladder. Bile salts act like laundry detergent, emulsifying lipid molecules. This process breaks down the lipid and exposes more surface to the effects of the digestive enzyme, lipase. Ultimately, short chains of fatty acids separated from this solution.

Bile salts are not normally excreted from the body. They are recycled. Once their work (emulsifying lipid molecules) is complete, they are reabsorbed from the intestine, recycled by the liver, and returned to the gallbladder for future use. This occurs through a closed system of blood vessels known as the portal system. Bile acid does not usually escape this system in a healthy dog.

The digestion of lipids takes one more odd turn. Instead of being absorbed directly into the blood stream, as are sugars and amino acids, fatty acids are taken up by the **lymphatic system**. Since the primary role of the lymphatic system is to the fight infection, lipid digestion is really a secondary role to immune system function. Ultimately, however, lipids are dumped into the blood stream and circulated to offer the body a concentrated source of energy. ✱

Chapter 4

Diabetes Mellitus

Abnormal Canine Metabolism — Diabetes

In the diabetic dog, metabolism does not take place as described in Chapter 3. Blood glucose levels can range from 130 mg/dl to 400 mg/dl, or more. The pancreas produces defective or insufficient insulin or it produces no insulin at all. In these cases, glucose cannot enter the cells. So even though large amounts of glucose are present in the bloodstream, the cells are still hungry. They begin to starve. This may cause a dog to have signs of weakness, depression, or lethargy.

Unable to obtain glucose, the starving cells send several inappropriate messages to the brain. The first message fools the brain into releasing glycogen from the liver. This is why a diabetic's blood glucose level may be high even when he is not eating. A second message tells the dog's brain to increase his appetite (known as **polyphagia**). This is why your dog may seem hungrier than usual. A third message tells the brain to break down the tissues of the dog's own body (muscle protein and body fat) into sugar.

All of these are emergency attempts to provide the cells with food. Unfortunately, they are futile. Without insulin, all the glucose in the world cannot reach the cells. The result: uncontrolled diabetics often exhibit two very contradictory symptoms. They have ravenous appetites while they simultaneously lose weight. Some dogs begin to behave aggressively when food is present. Such symptoms will dissipate once this disease is properly treated.

If *not* properly treated, the body's protective mechanisms can actually begin to cause the dog harm. As the body converts body fat into glucose, it produces by-products known as ketone acids or **ketones**. These accumulate in the blood stream, making the blood highly acidic. This state is known as **ketoacidosis**.

While these acids will eventually be excreted in the urine (called **ketonuria**) ketones can cause severe metabolic problems. Ketoacidosis may result in dehydration, racing pulse and respiration, vomiting, seizures, coma, or death. Thankfully, most dogs are diagnosed and treated long before this stage occurs.

There can be other complications of diabetes, as well. Since glucose cannot enter the cells, excess amounts accumulate in the blood stream. This is known as having high blood sugar or **hyperglycemia.** Consistently high levels, over time, can result in nerve and organ damage throughout the dog's body. To reduce the chance of damage, the body initiates another set of protective measures.

When the glucose level reaches a point where the kidneys can no longer process it (known as the **renal threshold**), the body will attempt to flush out the excess by dumping it into the urine. Sugar in the urine is known as **glucosuria** and is actually how the disease earned its name. "Diabetes" comes from a Greek word meaning "to siphon" and "mellitus" comes from a Latin word meaning "sweet like honey" (referring to the glucose).

In another protective measure, a message is sent to the brain to increase urinary frequency. This results in another common sign of diabetes: increased urination or **polyuria.** Dog owners report increases in both the volume of urine and the frequency of accidents in the house.

Polyuria results in excessive excretion of **magnesium**, a mineral crucial to normal body function and metabolism. Magnesium deficiency is extremely common among human diabetics. Studies indicate that magnesium improves tissue (cell membrane) sensitivity to insulin.

Since more water is required to flush the glucose, the brain also tells the dog to drink more water. The result is **polydipsia** or excessive thirst. These problems will subside once the disease is under control. Until that time, it is important to have adequate water available for your dog. Do not withhold water in an attempt to reduce accidents in the house.

Even with excellent treatment, certain complications of diabetes are still common. Dogs may develop diabetic **cataracts** or **dry eye syndrome**. They may develop skin, bladder, or ear **infections**. And the function of other internal organs, such as the kidneys and liver, may be strained.

Finally, dogs that develop one hormonal illness have an increased tendency toward developing a second one. Such examples include **hypothyroidism** (insufficient thyroid hormone production) or **Cushing's disease** (a disease of excess cortisol production). Excess cortisol can mimic signs of diabetes. Examples include muscle weakness, polydipsia, and polyuria.

Types of Diabetes

In the past, various forms of diabetes mellitus (DM) were either classified by the patient's age at onset or by the method in which they were controlled. Examples include "juvenile onset," "adult onset," **insulin dependent** diabetes mellitus (IDDM), and **non-insulin dependent** diabetes mellitus (NIDDM). These terms are still in use, but more recently, diabetes cases are being classified by their cause.

Diabetes mellitus caused by the **destruction of pancreatic beta cells** is termed **Type 1 diabetes**. In these cases, there are insufficient functioning beta cells present to produce the necessary levels of insulin. Replacement insulin *must* be supplied for these patients by injection. These dogs are insulin dependent. Most dogs are diagnosed with Type 1 diabetes mellitus.

Type 2 diabetes is caused either by *defective* insulin molecules or by insulin resistance. In the latter, insulin is present, but the cell membranes or receptors resist the transfer of glucose. Gestational diabetes in dogs is included in this group. Hormones produced during pregnancy block the effects of insulin. Blood glucose levels usually return to normal after the puppies are delivered.

Type 2 diabetes can be controlled by diet and oral medications (pills). Oral medications assist insulin in crossing the cell membrane. In some cases, however, Type 2 can progress to a point where insulin injections are needed. So Type 2 diabetes can be *either* insulin dependent or non-insulin dependent. In general, Type 2 DM is more common in cats and is *uncommon* in dogs.

Diabetes insipidus is a rare disorder of water imbalance. The body is unable to concentrate urine. Diabetes insipidus is a completely different disease than diabetes mellitus and is beyond the scope of this book. Consequently, any time the word "diabetes" is used alone in this text, it refers to diabetes mellitus.

Causes of Diabetes

It is normal to wonder how a pet developed diabetes. Dog owners want to know how the choices they make affect their pets. They wonder if it is possible to avoid similar situations in the future. DM is presently considered to be an *autoimmune* disease.

Autoimmune Disease

Normally, the dog's immune system protects his body from invading organisms such as yeast, bacteria, and viruses. The immune system responds in a variety of ways to fight off and kill these invaders. In most cases, it is a marvelously successful system. In other cases, the immune response is faulty.

In faulty systems, the body can over-react to invaders and become confused into fighting its own cells and tissues. These are referred to as **immune-mediated conditions** or **autoimmune diseases.** (While there are slight differences in the meanings of these terms, most people use them interchangeably.) Symptoms can include extreme allergic reactions, chronic inflammation, irritation, or the destruction of one's own cells and tissues (hence the term "auto," meaning "self"). In cases of DM, the immune system destroys the body's own pancreatic beta cells. Without beta cells, the body cannot produce insulin.

Current theory suggests that there is a genetic component to the occurrence of autoimmune disease. There does seem to be a prevalence of DM within certain breeds. However, it is believed that environmental factors also play a role. While the *tendency* toward immune-mediated diseases may be genetically inherited, it takes something in the environment to trigger the disease. Consequently, it is difficult to predict the occurrence of DM in related dogs.

Contributing Factors

Diabetes involves many intricate systems of the body. Illness in one area can strongly influence another area. It is common for diabetes to develop in the presence of endocrine imbalances, such as Cushing's disease and thyroid disease. The opposite is also true. Diabetes can seemingly precipitate these conditions, as well.

A similar relationship exists between the endocrine pancreas (insulin production) and the exocrine pancreas (digestion). Diabetes is commonly preceded, or followed, by cases of pancreatitis or pancreatic insufficiency.

The veterinary literature commonly cites the following factors as contributing to cases of DM: viral infections, chronic pancreatitis, chronic small bowel inflammation, obesity, hyperadrenocorticism (Cushing's disease), and the long-term use of prescription steroids or progesterone drugs. In addition, there is one significant factor that has largely been ignored, and that is the dog's diet. (This is discussed in great detail in Chapter 7, *What Causes These Diseases?*)

Prevalence

Diabetes mellitus is typically a disease of middle-aged dogs. Onset frequently occurs between seven to nine years of age. Juvenile dogs do sometimes develop the disease, but it is less common.

A minor degree of controversy exists as to whether particular breeds are predisposed to DM. Most sources assert that there is such a link. The suspected breeds include Poodles, Beagles, Dachshunds, and Miniature Schnauzers.

Diagnosing Diabetes Mellitus

Your veterinarian may recommend several types of laboratory tests to get a clear picture of your dog's condition. The majority of these are accomplished from a simple blood drawing.

The **complete blood count** (or CBC) may prove essentially normal with the exception of increased white blood cells.

A **serum cholesterol and triglyceride concentration** test often indicates increased levels of lipids in the bloodstream. This is a common finding in untreated diabetics as the body breaks down body fat.

A **serum biochemical panel**, which measures liver function, may indicate increased levels of liver enzymes, especially alkaline phosphatase (abbreviated as ALKP, ALP or SAP). Some dogs demonstrate increased or abnormal levels of serum bile acid (circulating levels of bile acids) and increased serum bilirubin levels, as well.

Pancreatic enzyme tests may indicate generalized pancreatic disease, which often accompanies DM. Test results frequently include raised levels of amylase and lipase enzymes.

Urinalysis (analysis of urine) may offer the most consistent findings in cases of DM. These commonly include glucosuria (sugar in the urine), ketonuria (ketones in the urine), proteinuria (protein in the urine), and bacteriuria (bacteria in the urine.) ✳

Chapter 5

Cushing's Disease and Excess Cortisol Production

Hyperadrenocorticism (HAC) refers to a state of elevated ("hyper") adrenal cortisol ("adreno-cortico") levels. Dr. Harvey Cushing first described this condition in 1932. His patients exhibited chronic excesses of cortisol circulating in their bodies and were diagnosed as having **Cushing's disease**.

There are several different causes of hyperadrenocorticism. The term Cushing's disease specifically refers to those cases caused by a problem in the pituitary gland, but for our purposes, the terms Cushing's disease and hyperadrenocoricism may be used interchangeably, as Cushing's disease is the term with which most dog owners are familiar.

Abnormal Canine Metabolism — Cushing's Disease

Since cortisol affects nearly every cell in the body, an excess of cortisol results in a wide variety of symptoms. This variety of symptoms is known as a syndrome. Consequently, some veterinarians refer to this situation as Cushing's syndrome or more specifically canine Cushing's syndrome.

Whichever term is used, the underlying problem remains the same. Too much cortisol or cortisone (a synthetic steroid) is circulating through the dog's body. In most cases, excess cortisol production stems from a malfunction of the pituitary gland, at the base of the brain. In some cases, it may stem from a problem of the adrenal glands, located near the kidneys. In other cases, Cushing's disease is induced by the use of prescription steroids.

Cortisol's primary job is to ensure the presence of glucose in the bloodstream. It does this by balancing the effects of insulin during carbohydrate metabolism. Whereas insulin helps mobilize glucose into hungry cells and *out of* the bloodstream, cortisol does almost the opposite. Cortisol helps mobilize glucose back *into* the bloodstream by breaking down muscle and adipose (fat) tissue.

When excess cortisol is present, though, it breaks down far too much muscle tissue (**catabolism**), causing **muscle weakness** and wasting. This can affect the dog's skeletal muscles with signs of fatigue, lethargy, or reduced coordination. Cortisol can also weaken other muscles, such as the heart, causing cardiac irregularities, murmurs, and congestive heart failure. It can weaken the bladder wall and sphincter muscles, causing urinary incontinence and dribbling. It can affect dental health by weakening ligaments in the gums.

When the body breaks down adipose tissue (**lipolysis**) it raises levels of cholesterol and tryglicerides circulating in the bloodstream. Catabolism and lipolysis are the same processes that occur during periods of starvation. Believing this to be the case, the appetite center of the brain erroneously tells the dog to eat more. So, despite the fact that Cushinoid dogs have sufficient levels of circulating glucose and ravenous appetites, they still feel hungry. This is known as **polyphagia** (excess hunger).

Catabolism can also cause dramatic rises in blood glucose levels, particularly in stressful situations. Dogs that are simultaneously diabetic may require higher levels of insulin to handle the rise in glucose. This scenario is sometimes referred to as **insulin resistance**, but it may also be described as simply a greater *need* for insulin. Excess cortisol can cause a once-regulated diabetic to become uncontrolled and can cause dog owners much frustration.

Cushinoid dogs are more susceptible to infection since excess cortisol **depresses the immune system**. This includes both the production and function of white blood cells. Pathogens reproduce more freely and attack the body. Skin, ear, and urinary tract infections are *commonly* seen in these dogs.

Cortisol normally regulates kidney function. Excess adrenal gland activity may result in the retention of sodium (and a rise in blood pressure). Cortisol increases the filtration rate, causing excessive urination (**polyuria**), and excessive drinking (**polydipsia**). Polyuria, in turn, causes excessive excretion of **magnesium**, a mineral crucial to normal body function and metabolism. Without magnesium, calcium can not be deposited into skeletal bone. Instead, high levels of calcium remain circulating in the bloodstream.

Cushinoid dogs commonly experience **heat intolerance.** These dogs pant excessively and seek cool surfaces to dissipate their body heat. This problem can stem from two factors. First, excess cortisol raises metabolic rate and body temperature in an attempt to kill perceived invaders. Second, a scenario is created in which magnesium levels are deficient and cortisol levels are in excess. This results in **potassium** being moved out of the cells, into the bloodstream, and excreted by urination. (Magnesium normally maintains potassium *inside* the cells and sodium in the fluid *around* the cells.) Potassium loss results in symptoms of fatigue and heat exhaustion.

Calcium and phosphorus levels are normally maintained at a 2:1 ratio in the body. When levels of serum phosphorus are high, the body tries to maintain the normal ratio by raising levels of serum calcium. To achieve this, the body increases parathyroid gland activity (hyperparathyroidism), and secretes hyperparathyroid hormone. This activity pulls calcium from the intestinal tract, or from skeletal bones and cartilage (known as demineralization). This scenario may contribute to joint and bone pain (limping) and collapsed tracheal cartilage.

In these cases, calcium may also be deposited into the body's soft tissues. Such areas include the skin (resulting in itchy sores known as calcinosis cutis), the lungs, bladder (calcium stones), skeletal joints (resulting in signs of arthritis) and, some experts believe, the corneal and lens tissues of the eye.

Cortisol is normally involved in the maintenance of the body's soft connective tissues. Excess cortisol disrupts the structure of elastic tissue under the skin and mucous membranes. This results in thinning of the hair and skin, cracked noses, and a loose, pendulous appearance to the dog's abdomen.

Chronic excesses of cortisol cause lesions to develop on the liver. Such liver disease can raise levels of circulating liver enzymes.

Cortisol is involved in the normal function of the nervous system. Excess cortisol and insufficient magnesium levels negatively affect cognitive function, resulting in a condition sometimes described as canine cognitive disorder. Signs can include mood changes such as depression, aggression, stupor, hearing impairment, and confusion (circling).

Cushinoid dogs are more susceptible to epileptic seizures. Opinions are split as to the reason behind this. Some experts believe that excess cortisol and insufficient magnesium lower the tolerance level toward seizure activity. Others believe that pituitary tumors place pressure on areas of the brain and initiate seizure activity.

Related to nervous system function is that of ophthalmic function. Cushioned dogs (and sub-clinical Cushioned dogs) sometimes experience dry eye syndrome, uveitis, or sudden blindness. (See Chapter 12, *Additional Health Concerns* for more details on these conditions.)

Under normal conditions, cortisol levels follow a seasonal and circadian rhythm (a 24-hour pattern) in humans and most other mammals. Levels are normally highest during the daytime and lowest at night. Cortisol has an inverse relationship to another hormone called melatonin. Melatonin is produced by the pineal gland, deep within the brain, and is considered to be responsible for the waking and sleeping patterns of a normal circadian rhythm.

Melatonin levels are normally lowest during the daylight and highest as darkness falls. As levels increase, so does drowsiness. In some cases of hyperadrenocorticism, excess cortisol seems to disrupt this cycle. Many dogs may sleep during the day and experience varying degrees of **insomnia** during the night. Some dogs are simply **agitated**. Others retire, only to wake their owners repeatedly during the night. Insufficient levels of magnesium also contribute to increased irritability and insomnia.

Types of Hyperadrenocorticism

There are three basic types of hyperadrenocorticism: pituitary-dependent, adrenal-dependent, and iatrogenic.

Pituitary-dependent

The vast majority of cases in dogs, 80% to 90%, are classified as pituitary-dependent hyperadrenocorticism (PDH). Pituitary-dependent means the problem lies within the pituitary gland located near the brain. Most often this involves a pituitary tumor that excretes excessive adrenocorticotrophic hormone (ACTH). The excess ACTH sends a constant message to the adrenal glands to produce cortisol. This chronic demand causes the adrenal glands to become enlarged.

Adrenal-dependent

The second type of hyperadrenocorticism is classified as adrenal-dependent or adreno-cortical-dependent. "Adreno" refers to the adrenal glands; "cortico" refers to the layer of the gland (the cortex) that produces cortisol. As the name implies, these cases involve a problem of the adrenal glands, usually a cortisol-secreting tumor on one or the other of the glands.

About 15% to 20% of all hyperadrenocorticism cases are classified as adrenal tumors (ATs). Of these, about one-half are malignant; the other half are not. Adrenal tumors secrete cortisol independent of ACTH control. The high levels of cortisol shut off the pituitary release of ACTH. This causes the non-cancerous adrenal gland to stop production of cortisol and to atrophy or waste away.

Iatrogenic Hyperadrenocorticism

The third classification of this disease is known as iatrogenic hyperadrenocorticism. These cases result when the dog is treated with long-term or high doses of glucocorticoids, also known as steroids, such as prednisone or cortisone or their derivatives. In these cases, the body believes that sufficient levels of cortisol are present and reduces its production of ACTH. No longer required to work, the adrenal glands atrophy.

Causes of Hyperadrenocorticism

In cases of iatrogenic HAC, the source of the problem is known to be therapeutic administration of cortisol. The veterinary literature does not provide a clearcut cause for pituitary-dependant HAC and adrenal tumors. In humans, there is some evidence that a genetic predisposition exists toward these conditions.

Contributing Factors

Hyperadrenocorticism involves many intricate systems of the body. Illness in one area of the body can strongly influence another area. One example of this is the relationship between Cushing's disease and other metabolic/endocrine/immune disorders. It is common for Cushing's to develop in the presence of diabetes, pancreatitis, and bowel disease. The opposite is also true. Cushing's disease can seemingly precipitate these conditions, as well. In addition, there is one significant factor that has largely been ignored, and that is the dog's diet. (This is discussed in great detail in Chapter 7, *What Causes These Diseases?*)

Prevalence

Cushing's disease is most often diagnosed in obese, middle-aged dogs of six years or more. Atypically, however, it can occur in dogs as young as one year of age. There is some discussion as to predisposition by sex, but this is arguable. Some sources indicate a higher incidence of adrenal tumor in female dogs.

The same puzzle applies to predisposition by breed. Some sources argue that none exists, while others report that the Boxer, Boston Terrier, Dachshund, Beagle, Yorkshire Terrier and Miniature Poodle are at higher risk for pituitary-dependent hyperadrenocorticism.

Diagnosing Cushing's Disease

A variety of diagnostic tests are available to confirm cases of HAC and differentiate their causes. Your veterinarian may chose one particular test or procedure over another to determine the most appropriate therapy and accurate prognosis for your dog.

These tests are not, however, 100% accurate. Numerous factors can contribute to the interpretation of the test results. Since the immune system responds to a vast number of stressors with the release of cortisol, the tests can easily be skewed by psychological stress, chronic illness (diabetes, inflammatory bowel syndrome, etc.), steroid use, or exhaustion of the glands, themselves.

The best veterinarians look at the entire picture when diagnosing Cushing's disease and problems of excess cortisol production. This includes physical signs and findings, the owners observations, and blood cell counts, in addition to Cushing's tests. Many dogs exhibit clinical signs of excess cortisol without ever truly testing positive for Cushing's disease. Tests are commonly repeated when results are questionable.

ACTH Stimulation Test

This test is considered by many veterinarians to be the best initial test for diagnosing the presence of hyperadrenocorticism. It is relatively simple, quick, and cost-effective. It operates on the theory that when a normal dog is given ACTH by injection, the adrenal glands will be stimulated to produce cortisol.

It can be used to distinguish whether HAC is a result of iagtrogenic or natural causes. It is *not* good at diagnosing between pituitary-dependent and adrenal-dependent cases and it is not always recommended in cases of concurrent illness, such as diabetes or renal failure.

The veterinarian will likely perform this test before starting the dog on medication. It provides important "before and after" information about the levels of ACTH and cortisol in the dog's system. It is important to discontinue any steroid medications (prednisone and its derivatives) the dog is receiving several weeks to months before this test is administered.

The majority of dogs both with pituitary-dependent and adrenal-dependent HAC will demonstrate an exaggerated rise in cortisol levels after the ACTH injection (greater than about 20 ug/dl (U.S.) or 550 mmol/l (Canada)). Little or no rise in post-test cortisol levels is called a "flat-line" result and is suggestive of iatrogenic causes.

To complicate matters even further, a normal response to the ACTH stimulation test does not rule out Cushing's disease! Between 5% and 20% of dogs that *do* have HAC will not demonstrate the expected rise in cortisol after the ACTH injection.

The ACTH test is often performed first thing in the morning after the dog has fasted overnight. It involves drawing a pre-injection blood sample, called a **resting cortisol level**, which is followed by the intravenous injection of synthetic ACTH. The dosage is specific to the dog's weight. One to two hours later, the dog's blood is drawn to measure the level of circulating cortisol. Greater than normal rises in cortisol levels indicate Cushing's disease.

Some veterinarians keep the dog in the clinic during this time, others permit the owner to sit with the dog on the clinic grounds or direct the owner to return at the designated time. In reality, the latter may actually be less stress ful for the dog, resulting in a more accurate test result.

The ACTH stimulation test will periodically be repeated to assess your dog's responsiveness to medical treatment. (See pages 125-126, *Lysodren,* for a further discussion of ACTH testing.) This may vary from 3- to 6-month intervals. If test results are inconclusive, the test may be repeated, or a more extensive test may be recommended.

Once hyperadrenocorticism has been diagnosed, the next step is to differentiate the cause, that is, determine whether the problem stems from the pituitary or adrenal glands. This knowledge will help the veterinarian develop a treatment plan. Dexamethosone Suppression Tests are the next step in making this differentiation.

Low Dose Dexamethasone Suppression (LDDS) Test

The LDDS test is helpful as a "second opinion" when a veterinarian finds results of the ACTH stimulation test questionable. The LDDS test also helps differentiate between cases of pituitary-dependent disease and adrenal-dependent disease.

The LDDS procedure also involves drawing a pre-injection blood sample to measure the resting cortisol level. This is followed by the intravenous administration of a low dose of dexamethasone, a cortisone-type drug. The dog's blood will be drawn at four and eight hours later and will again measure cortisol levels. The dog will usually be hospitalized during this period.

In *normal* dogs the pituitary gland responds to the presence of dexamethasone by shutting off the feedback loop between the adrenal and pituitary glands. In other words, dexamethasone normally suppresses both cortisol and ACTH production. As a result, circulating levels of cortisol will slowly decline over an 8-hour period. In Cushinoid dogs, the body does not respond in the normal way. The abnormal response can help differentiate HAC cases in the follow ways:

In cases of **adrenal tumors**, when cortisol is secreted independently of ACTH control, the dexamethasone may not affect cortisol levels but may, instead, lower the levels of circulating ACTH. However, these responses can vary considerably, making the test results difficult to interpret.

In cases of **pituitary-dependent** HAC, the tumor ignores low doses of dexamethasone. Cortisol levels do not drop. In fact, the test may even indicate an increase in cortisol levels.

Unfortunately, the LDDS test may result in false positives more than half of the time. Results of the LDDS test are particularly susceptible to the effects of stress. These can include the emotional stress of simply going to the veterinary clinic, or the physical stress of chronic disease.

High Dose Dexamethasone Suppression (HDDS) Test

The HDDS test is more helpful in differentiating cases of pituitary-dependent and adrenal-dependent HAC. *High doses* of dexamethasone can suppress ACTH/ cortisol production in most pituitary-dependant dogs. As with the low-dose test, this procedure involves intravenous injection of dexamethasone, and an in-hospital stay of eight hours. If the post-injection level of cortisol is less than 50% of the pre-injection level, PDH is suspected.

Dogs with adrenal tumors do not suppress cortisol levels even after high doses of dexamethasone are injected. A small percentage of dogs are resistant to this test.

Combination Dexamethasone Suppression and ACTH Stimulation Test

This test diagnoses Cushing's disease but does not reliably differentiate pituitary-dependent disease from adrenal-dependent disease.

Additional tests:

The **Urinary Cortisol Creatinine Ratio Test (UCCR)**

This test measures cortisol levels in the urine. It is used as an *indication* of Cushing's disease and usually requires substantiation by a more specific Cushing's test.

The **Endogenous ACTH Test**

This is a one-time, specially processed measurement of the body's own ACTH production. In cases of pituitary-dependent HAC, ACTH levels will be high. In cases of adrenal-dependent HAC, ACTH levels will be low.

Radiographs (or X-rays) and **Ultrasound Examination**

Both of these tests are helpful in determining the size of the liver and the adrenal glands, if they are calcified. Calcification occurs in about 30% of adrenal tumors. Radiographs may also demonstrate other problems of calcium metabolism, including demineralization (bone thinning) and calcification of soft tissues, such as lungs, bronchi and bladder. ✳

Chapter 6

Pancreatic Disease

The suffix "-itis" literally means "inflammation." Pancreatitis refers to inflammation of the pancreas. If your dog has been diagnosed with diabetes mellitus, you are already familiar with the insulin-producing portion of the pancreas or **endocrine pancreas**. This chapter will examine some of the diseases of the **exocrine pancreas**, the portion that produces digestive enzymes.

Abnormal Canine Metabolism – Pancreatic Disease

When the pancreas is under significant stress, either by overwork or irritation, it becomes inflamed. The adrenal glands may release cortisol to help reduce this inflammation, but ultimately, the tissues of the pancreas swell and obstruct the pancreatic duct. This causes digestive enzymes to accumulate within the pancreas. The high concentration of enzymes overwhelms the system that normally maintains them in their inactive state. As this protective system fails, enzymes become active while still in the pancreas. Auto-digestion, scarring, and further inflammation are the results.

Pancreatic inflammation can result in varying degrees of pain. This can range from mild discomfort upon abdominal palpitation to severe pain requiring prescription medication. When some dogs experience pain, they lose their appetite. When the pain is resolved, their interest in food usually returns.

Foods are poorly digested when digestive enzymes cannot reach the small intestine. The dog's body may consider these incompletely digested molecules to be toxins or irritants. This is particularly true of dietary protein. The body often regards large protein molecules as invading organisms, which can initiate an immune system response.

Digestion of dietary fats (lipids) can be particularly compromised in cases of pancreatitis. There are several likely reasons for this. Prematurely activated enzymes can enter the lymphatic system and travel to the liver, causing tissue damage. The close proximity of the pancreas to the liver can result in inflammation of liver tissue and bile duct. This can interfere with both the production and secretion of **bile**. If sufficient amounts of bile are unable to reach the small intestine, dietary lipids will not be completely digested.

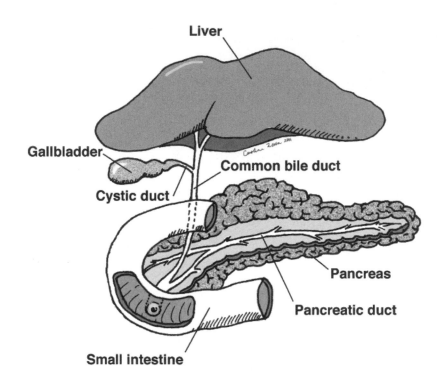

Unlike sugars and amino acids that are absorbed into the bloodstream, fatty acids are absorbed into the **lymphatic system**. Since the primary role of the lymphatic system is immune response, its role in handling lipid digestion is really secondary to its role in defending the body. If the dog's body is fighting infection or inflammation, lipid digestion will be compromised. Consequently, the dog's stools may be coated with undigested lipids, resulting in a greasy appearance.

The body also attempts to protect itself by speeding these irritants out of the gastrointestinal tract. This can be accomplished in either of two ways. Food in the stomach can be expelled by deep contractions of the abdomen and diaphragm — **vomiting**. Partially digested food in the small intestine can be removed by rapid contraction of the intestinal tract. While this action does speed irritants out of the body, it interferes with the normal water absorption in the bowel. This results in loose stools or **diarrhea**. In severe cases, vomiting and diarrhea can result in potassium loss. This can upset the acid/alkaline relationship of the body.

Despite these aggressive attempts to rid the body of digestive irritants, they are not always successful. In these dogs it is common to see **inflammatory bowel disease** or malabsorption conditions concurrent with cases of pancreatitis. Dogs with absorption problems may have difficulty reabsorbing bile salts from the small intestine and may experience periodic vomiting of bile, a frothy, yellow fluid. These dogs may also have difficulty absorbing oral medications and dietary minerals such as magnesium and calcium.

Types of Pancreatitis

Pancreatic disease follows few hard, fast rules. A dog may experience a single episode of pancreatitis once in his lifetime or frequent episodes that may return repeatedly. Cases of pancreatitis can be so mild that they resolve themselves in a few hours. They can also be so severe as to be life threatening.

When inflammation occurs gradually and over time it is termed **chronic pancreatitis**. This form of the disease is most common in dogs. Chronic inflammation may result in scarring (fibrosis) and permanent damage to the pancreas. Inflammation can affect the surrounding organs and tissue. This includes the insulin-producing portion of the pancreas, as well as the liver.

In other cases, the inflammation is sudden and severe. This is termed **acute pancreatitis**. It has a more sudden onset, but does not last as long as cases of chronic pancreatitis. Acute cases are also less common than chronic cases.

Signs of acute pancreatitis can include vomiting, abdominal pain, loss of appetite, and diarrhea. These dogs may also exhibit alterations in activity levels. They may be restless *or* unwilling to move about. Other signs can include depression, weakness, and irritability. These signs may also indicate potassium deficiency. Not all dogs will exhibit all signs. Cases of chronic pancreatitis can present more subtle signs. They may only appear intermittently or to a slight degree.

Complications of acute pancreatitis can include liver problems such as disseminated intravascular coagulation (DIC), a serious blood-clotting abnormality. Inflammation can compromise the liver's ability to process bilirubin, which results in jaundice. Cysts and abscesses of the pancreas can develop after acute episodes of pancreatitis. Kidney failure, fluid around the lungs, diabetes mellitus, heart arrhythmia, and shock are additional considerations.

Upon examination, dogs may exhibit high levels of white blood cells circulating in the bloodstream. Levels of amylase and lipase are often, but not always, high. Kidney function tests may also be elevated.

Other Pancreatic Diseases

Pancreatic Exocrine Insufficiency (PEI) (also called Exocrine Pancreatic Insufficiency)

This condition is a separate from pancreatitis. It is included in this discussion, however, because of its probable connection with the other ailments covered in this book.

Pancreatic insufficiency represents an inability to produce sufficient amounts of digestive enzymes. In some cases, there appears to be an inherited condition. In other cases it is linked to the damage sustained by chronic pancreatitis. Scarred areas of the exocrine pancreas are unable to produce enzymes. But in most cases, the cells that produce enzymes simply atrophy or waste away.

Signs of PEI include chronic diarrhea and weight loss despite a good, even ravenous appetite. This healthy appetite is due to the fact that nutrients are poorly absorbed. The appetite center in the brain is never satisfied and continues to send the dog a message of hunger. These dogs may also experience malabsorption problems, inflammatory bowel disease, or colitis, worsened by the presence of undigested foods.

Causes of Pancreatitis

The veterinary community admits to being unsure as to the exact cause of pancreatitits. It does appear, though, that prior to the onset of full-blown pancreatitis (auto-digestion), the pancreas is already inflamed.

Contributing Factors

Illness in one area of the body can strongly influence another area. One example of this is the relationship between pancreatitis and other metabolic/endocrine/immune disorders. It is common for pancreatitis to develop in the presence of liver problems, Cushing's disease, or chronic bowel disease. The opposite is also true. Pancreatitis can seemingly precipitate these conditions, as well.

A similar relationship exists between the exocrine pancreas (digestion) and the endocrine pancreas (insulin production). Pancreatitis is commonly preceded, or followed, by cases of diabetes.

The veterinary literature points toward the following factors in the development of pancreatitis: diets high in fat content, obesity, Cushing's disease, and the use of prescription corticosteroids. There has also been one contributing factor that has been largely overlooked, and that is the dog's diet. (This is discussed in great detail in Chapter 7, *What Causes These Diseases?*)

Prevalence

Pancreatitis appears to be a disease of overweight and middle-aged dogs. There also seems to be a predisposition of certain breeds. This includes Cockers Spaniels, Miniature Schnauzers, and Miniature Poodles. German Shepherd Dogs seem especially prone to PEI.

Diagnosing Pancreatic Disease

Veterinarians use several blood tests to diagnose pancreatitis. These tests generally measure **levels of enzymes** present in the bloodstream. One enzyme used to evaluate pancreatic inflammation is amylase; another is lipase. Some doctors believe that the lipase test is more indicative, but neither test is entirely accurate. In some cases, enzymes may be present due to other disease processes. And some dogs *with* pancreatitis never exhibit elevated levels of either enzyme.

A third blood test used to diagnose pancreatitis is known as the **trypsinogen-like-immunoreactivity** (or TLI) **test.** This test measures trypsin and trypsinogen, two enzymes in the protease family. The TLI test is more reliable than previous enzyme tests and it is especially helpful in diagnosing cases of *acute* pancreatitis and pancreatic enzyme insufficiency. Unfortunately, it is only performed at a limited number of laboratories, and it may require two weeks time to receive the test results.

Additional diagnostic findings may include elevated **levels of white blood cells** (WBCs). Doctors may also suggest abdominal x-rays, ultrasound procedures, or needle biopsies. These procedures are not 100% accurate in diagnosis, either. ✻

Chapter 7

What Causes These Diseases?

Life is more hectic, urban, and commercial than it was thirty or forty years ago. This has clearly been reflected in how we feed ourselves and our dogs. We embrace convenience. Unfortunately, convenient, commercial diets seem to play a major role in the development of canine DM, Cushing's disease, pancreatitis, inflammatory bowel disease, kidney and liver disease, and skin allergies.

Commercial Diets

Commercial diets are exactly that, those that can be commercially purchased at retail stores or veterinary clinics. Most Americans feed their dogs commercial foods, and most veterinarians support that decision.

Under the heading of commercial dog food, there exist several different categories. The first will be referred to as supermarket dog food. These are the canned, semi-moist, and dry (kibble) foods that are available at supermarkets, grocery stores, and warehouses.

The next category includes prescription dog foods. These are only available through veterinary clinics. They are produced in both canned and dry formulas and are tailored toward specific digestion problems, such as kidney disease, bowel inflammation, etc. There are even a few designed specifically toward controlling blood glucose levels.

Additionally, there are some commercial diets that are advertised as "premium" food. Available as canned food and kibble, these diets typically contain more consistent ingredients from one batch to the next. They are available at large chain pet-supply stores, but never at grocery stores.

Finally, there are increasing numbers of natural or holistic pet foods. These are available in canned, kibble, and even frozen formulas. They can be found at holistic and high-end pet supply shops, holistic veterinary clinics, and over the Internet.

The Benefits of Feeding Commercial Pet Foods

Many veterinarians will recommend prescription or premium dog foods for their patients suffering from DM, obesity, pancreatitis, and kidney disease. This may include an ever-growing selection of high-fiber, low-fat, and low-protein formulations. Different veterinarians have their personal favorites, as do dog's and their owners.

The traditional veterinary literature recommends feeding diabetic dogs a diet high in complex carbohydrates (grains) and fiber. These elements are thought to slow the absorption of glucose into the bloodstream. They are cited as preventing drastic swings in postprandial (after eating) glucose levels.

Commercial diets provide diabetic dogs with a fairly consistent type and amount of food. When a dog consumes a controlled number of daily calories, it is easier to determine an appropriate insulin dose.

Obese dogs and those with pancreatitis are frequently switched to low-fat diets. Most veterinarians believe that obesity and pancreatitis are closely linked. Accordingly, they recommend low-fat diets for these dogs, combined with gradual exercise programs to reduce weight.

Commercial diets are convenient for the dog owner. Dispensing a measured amount of kibble or canned food keeps mealtime uncomplicated. A simple feeding regime may reduce the chance of a pet owner feeling overwhelmed by his dog's disease.

Those are the benefits to feeding commercial food. As more literature becomes available regarding the role of diet in healthcare, however, it is valuable to examine more closely the content and effects of commercial diets. Following are a number of interesting findings. Some of them are newly published; others have been around for some time.

The Drawbacks of Feeding Commercial Pet Foods

To best understand this discussion, it is important to examine the physical design of the dog and what food is most appropriate to him. Some people believe that domestic dogs have adapted, anatomically, to their environment. They believe that over time the dog's digestive system has radically changed from that of his ancestor, the wolf. Most canine nutritionists disagree. They support the concept that dogs still maintain the inner workings of the wolf. Since there is much evidence to support this concept, let us begin here and consider the diet of the wild dog or wolf.

Paleontologists estimate that a period of approximately 100,000 years is required before evolutionary changes occur within a species. The most accepted theories estimate that dogs began their association with humans between 10,000 and 15,000 years ago. This is a much shorter time span than that considered necessary for evolutionary changes.

Dogs and wolves are physically very similar. Their DNA differs by only 1% to 2%. Humans have certainly manipulated the superficial appearance of the dog through selective breeding, but have not altered the dog's basic digestive workings at all.

Dogs and wolves are designed, *primarily,* to eat meat. They may scavenge many things, but their anatomy reveals much about which foods are, and are not, appropriate to them. Examine their teeth and jaws. They are designed for grasping and tearing meat. Dogs quickly gulp their food. This is quite different from herbivores and some omnivores that have broad, flat teeth designed for leisurely chewing.

As another comparison, human saliva contains amylase, an enzyme that aids in digestion. Amylase begins to break down carbohydrates during mastication (chewing). No digestive enzymes are present in the dog's saliva. Canine digestion does not begin until food reaches the stomach.

In addition to being a meat eater, the dog is also a scavenger. If something smells edible to him, and he is given the opportunity, a dog will eat almost anything. This includes decaying carcasses and animal droppings.

Depending on locale, a springtime diet of the wolf may include the eggs of waterfowl, young hatchlings, fish, and small birds. Summertime may bring a diet of rodents, pheasant, wild turkey, green vegetation, and fallen fruit. In autumn, many of today's wolves find injured deer or piles of innards left behind by human hunters. Large prey is frequently hidden or buried to be finished at a later time. Winter is a fight for whatever can be found.

Dogs are physically and metabolically designed to eat these foods. They possess very strong stomach acids and short digestive tracts. Many nutritionists believe that together, these protect the dog from numerous and ever-present germs in his environment. (Remember: dogs frequently eat and roll in feces and decayed carcasses as part of their normal behavior.) Bacteria are either killed in the stomach or hastened through the system before they can have any effect on the animal. The dog was designed to digest his meal *rapidly.*

With that history in mind, it is interesting to note how radically a typical commercial diet disagrees with the canine design. The topic of protein is as a good a place as any to begin this discussion.

Protein Sources in Commercial Foods

Most dog owners consider the term protein to mean meat. Grains also supply protein in the diet, and they will be discussed in a later section. Here, we will examine meat and its by-products.

In most commercial dog food, the meats being used have been declared "unfit for human consumption." Occasionally, it is possible to find a commercial pet food that contains high quality, human-grade meat, but this is rare and proudly advertised when it is the case. The meats found in most commercial dog food are, in essence, **the waste products** of the slaughterhouse industry. They are euphemistically referred to as the "4-Ds," livestock that is diseased, disabled, dead, or in the process of dying on its way to slaughter.

Meat by-products, meat by-product-meal, and bone meal are other phrases that disguise non-nutritious waste products. Meat rendering plants that produce these products may use any of the following ingredients in the rendering process:

> Diseased companion animals euthanized at veterinary clinics
> and shelters;
> Road-kill animals;
> Zoo animals dead from cancer and infection;
> Restaurant grease and garbage;
> Supermarket meats long past their expiration dates; and
> Cancerous tissue and tumors cut away from carcasses

These ingredients are cooked at high heats (greater than 170 degrees F.) This accomplishes two things. It helps preserve the food by destroying certain natural chemicals in the meat called enzymes and it permanently alters the arrangement of amino acids, the basic building blocks of protein.

Enzymes

There have been about 4,000 enzymes identified throughout nature. They fall into three major classes: metabolic enzymes, digestive enzymes, and food enzymes. All three are designed to work together in a beautifully balanced system.

Metabolic enzymes are present in the blood, tissues, and organs of the body. For example, white blood cells carry protease, the enzyme that digests protein. This enzyme is released against invading organisms as part of the immune system response.

Other examples of metabolic enzymes include liver enzymes and cardiac enzymes. These enzymes are responsible for cell growth and repair in their respective organs. Damage to the liver or heart can result in a release of enzymes into the bloodstream. You may have heard your own doctor or veterinarian discuss "elevated cardiac enzymes" or "elevated liver enzymes" such as alkaline phosphatase.

Digestive enzymes are those that the body produces to break down food items into useable nutrients. In the canine body, the stomach produces protease to digest protein. The exocrine portion of the pancreas produces additional protease, as well as amylase (to digest carbohydrates) and lipase (to digest fats/lipids).

Finally, there are enzymes present in all fresh food. They contribute to the breakdown of food (fermentation) when it is not preserved by chemicals or cooking. Nature's great design makes these available so the pancreas does not have to provide all of the necessary enzymes alone. While a minor degree of controversy exists on this topic, several studies indicate that **food enzymes** will digest 5% to75% of the food itself, without the help of the pancreas.

While some foods (starches) are made more digestible by cooking, most are not. High temperatures (usually 138 to 170 degrees F.) destroy the intrinsic enzymes in fresh foods, causing the pancreas to work harder. Over a lifetime, the pancreas has trouble keeping pace with the continual demands of a processed diet. Eventually, it may be unable to produce a sufficient quantity of enzymes. This may help explain why diseases of the pancreas are often seen in older dogs.

When the pancreas can no longer produce the necessary volume of enzymes, the body calls upon *metabolic* enzymes to aid in digestion. These stores can be found in the liver, spleen, kidneys, heart, and lungs. Enzymes are routed from these organs, through the bloodstream, and into the intestines to help break down food. High levels of enzymes in the blood (particularly serum lipase) are a good indication that the pancreas is overworked and inflamed.

The body can also draw additional enzymes from the bloodstream itself. The white blood cells contain numerous enzymes, including protease. Usually, this is used to attack invading organisms (proteins), but it can be very successful in aiding digestion. Many dogs with digestive problems demonstrate high white-blood cell counts.

This backup mechanism does have a flaw, however. When white blood cells are occupied with food digestion, they are distracted from their primary work of protecting the body. Their ability to fight invaders is compromised. This may contribute to the frequent infections seen in diabetic and Cushinoid dogs.

A number of medical studies demonstrate that the pancreas enlarges in dogs eating only processed food. In human healthcare, it is fairly well accepted that when an enlarged organ is accompanied by excessive function, it becomes exhausted. Degeneration is usually the result.

Incidences of pancreatitis are constantly increasing. This suggests that dogs have *not* evolved to effectively digesting a diet of highly processed foods. If dogs had evolved to this state, the pancreas would be capable of meeting the great demand for digestive enzymes. Clearly it has not.

Altered Amino Acids

Cooking at high temperatures for long periods also alters the arrangement of amino acids. The greater the degree of cooking, the more the amino acid arrangement is altered. They become increasingly indigestible.

About half of the altered amino acids in commercial diets are unusable by the canine body. In humans, inadequate supplies of amino acids have been implicated in a host of ailments. This includes impaired central nervous system function, impaired endocrine system function, and cancer growth due to impaired immune system function.

Altered chains of amino acids are difficult for the body to break apart. This causes an even greater demand for digestive enzymes. Some doctors even believe that the body regards these aberrant protein molecules, not as food, but as foreign invaders.

Slowed Digestion

Insufficient food enzymes and altered amino acids have a similar effect on the dog. The pancreas is called upon to increase the production and secretion of digestive enzymes. This takes time, and significantly slows the rate of digestion. Wild dogs and wolves digest their meals in a matter of 4 or 5 hours. In contrast, it can 8 to 15 hours for commercial dog food to break down, clear the stomach, and pass through the small intestine.

During this extended period, chemicals and other impurities have ample time to irritate and inflame the intestinal wall. The canine GI system was not designed to handle this. It was designed to process food quickly. Prolonged digestion lays the groundwork for disaster.

Bioavailability

Protein that contains useless amino acids, chemicals, cancer cells from 4-D livestock, and no enzymes is considered to be poor quality protein. It is difficult for a dog to absorb and utilize such protein. Canine nutritionists describe these foods as having "poor bioavailability." Poorly digested protein results in an accumulation of serum phosphorus.

Commercial dog foods may be supplemented with *large amounts* of protein in an attempt to compensate for the poor bioavailability. The theory is that since a dog can only utilize a fraction of the poor-quality protein, adding more will meet his body's needs. Unfortunately, more of a bad thing doesn't make it better. The dog's body was never designed to filter out so many impurities.

Most dogs eating commercial diets do eventually experience some degree of kidney or liver disease. Since these organs filter waste products from the body, they are constantly at work when so many impurities are present. When the liver is ill, it is no longer able to filter chemicals and waste products from the bloodstream. Medications and hormones such as estrogen and cortisol build up in the body. Bilirubin accumulates and can cause jaundice.

The heavy burden and constant inflammation also reduce kidney function. Healthy tissue is replaced by scar tissue that can no longer filter urine. This creates a vicious cycle of further scarring and greater loss of function.

Consider, again, the diet of the wild dog. His diet consists of 50% to 70% meat and meaty bones. His body secretes protein-digesting enzymes in two locations. This supports the belief that the dog is designed to eat a diet rich in protein. Yet, many dog owners are led to believe that commercial diets consisting of only 20% protein are *too rich* for their dogs.

This conflict exists because the statistics printed on pet food labels reflect only how a food breaks down *chemically*. This is not a reflection of the food's bioavailability, that is, whether the body can actually use it. In the final analysis, it is much more likely that *poor quality* protein is responsible for kidney degeneration, rather than the *quantity* of protein.

Fiber in Commercial Foods

Peanut hulls, almond shells, empty grain hulls, and beet pulp can all be added to commercial food as fiber. Beet pulp is the dried residue of sugar beets, essentially just sugar, which the diabetic can do without. The hulls of nuts and grains are used as fillers. They are used in many "lite" or "diet" formulations of pet foods, constituting as much as 15% of the diet.

None of these elements are natural to the dog. And given a choice, a dog would probably not eat these things on his own. In fact, many dogs intelligently refuse to eat these diets. They may forage elsewhere (including gardens, garbage cans, and countertops) in an attempt to find the nutrients they crave.

Chemicals in Commercial Foods

In addition to cooking commercial pet food, manufacturers must add a variety of potent chemicals to preserve it. Some of these include BHT, BHA, and ethoxyquin. BHT and BHA are prohibited in human food since they are known to contribute to cancer. Ethoxyquin is essentially a pesticide/herbicide. Various industry sources label it, *"Caution — Poison"* and *"Toxic by ingestion."* It has been implicated in a number of autoimmune disorders, and need only be listed on the dog food label if it was added at the production plant. Ethoxyquin can be added by the feed grain mill or the rendering plant, and *never appear on the label.*

In addition to preservatives, inorganic and toxic dyes are added to commercial food. Red, yellow, and blue dyes turn the food from gray to a pleasing reddish brown color. Pleasing, that is, to humans. Dogs do not perceive color well, and color is not an issue in their eating habits. These chemicals are added so the *owner* will find the food appealing.

Binding agents are added to the food to create the shapes of burgers and kibble. Clay products may be added to produce consistent-looking stools. Other additives can include anti-caking agents, drying agents, texturizers, stabilizers, and thickeners. And while not chemicals, per se, refined sugar and fat may be added to make the food more palatable. *Over the past few decades*, the level of chemicals found in most commercial food has increased.

Grains and the Endocrine Pancreas

Most commercial diets are not well-suited to the dog's physical make up and metabolism. In other words, they are not "biologically appropriate." They are primarily made up of grain products.

Contemporary canine nutritionists explain that dogs do not process *complex* carbohydrates (grains) well. Studies demonstrate that unlike humans, dogs do not "carbo-load," that is, store up energy from meals high in complex carbohydrates. While human athletes successfully practice this technique, it results in an accumulation of lactic acid in dogs. (Lactic acid causes the muscular pain experienced after unaccustomed exercise.) This demonstrates a marked difference in how dogs process complex carbohydrates.

Dog food labels list ingredients by weight, not volume, so lightweight grains can constitute the bulk of the ingredients without appearing first on the list. These diets can contain as much as 65% corn, wheat, rice, oats, barley, soy, rye, or combinations or components, thereof.

As previously mentioned, the dog is not physically designed to process large amounts of grain. Some is usually tolerated, and certain dogs can even live long lives subsisting on a mainstay of grain, but the average dog does not.

The makers of premium and prescription dog foods advertise the use of high-quality, whole grains in their food. They say these provide an "excellent source of protein" for dogs. Large amounts of grain may be an appropriate source of protein for some species, but *not so* for animals primarily designed to eat meat.

And when whole grain *is* used in dog food, it has often been deemed unfit for human consumption due to mold, contaminants, or poor handling practices. Some brands reportedly contain damaged, spilled, and spoiled grain known as "the tail of the mill." This can include the hulls, chaff, straw, dust, dirt, and sand swept from the mill floor at the end of each week.

Canine teeth are designed for tearing and ripping, not grinding. Unlike some other animals, dogs' saliva contains no amylase, the enzyme to digest carbohydrates. This places an added burden on the pancreas to produce enzymes. Grains are heavily used in dog food, not because they are *beneficial* to dogs, but because they are economical and readily available fillers.

Over the past few decades, the proportion of grain in commercial food *has increased*. A number of veterinarians and canine nutritionists are now beginning to question the heavy inclusion of grain in the canine diet, especially when fed to young puppies. Experts are implicating grain in an increasing number of autoimmune diseases being diagnosed today. A review of the immune system will help explain why.

A Review of the Immune System

The body protects itself from infection with an intricate system of endocrine glands, hormones, and cells. When an invading organism (a virus, for example) enters the body, white blood cells respond by producing materials called antibodies. Antibodies read and remember the protein make up of the invader. They become programmed to attack that invader any time it is encountered it in the future. This is the principle upon which vaccines are based.

One important family of antibodies is the immunoglobulins. Named with letters of the alphabet, each immunoglobulin has a different role in the immune response. **Immunoglobulin A** (or IgA) is secreted in a thin, protective layer in the body's mucous membranes. It is found in body fluids such as tears and saliva, as well as in the lungs, urinary bladder, and the intestines. IgA is considered to be the body's first line of defense. Like a row of soldiers, IgA prevents invaders from passing through the intestinal wall and into the body.

During normal digestion, protein is broken down into short chains of amino acids. The body recognizes these *short* chains or small protein molecules as food sources, not invaders. These fragments are allowed to pass by the IgA antibodies and through the intestinal wall to provide nutrition. The body recognizes larger protein molecules as invaders. Normally, these molecules are too large to squeeze past the IgA antibodies.

In some instances, however, large proteins *are* able to infiltrate the intestinal wall. The first example is seen in young puppies, weaned from mother's milk as early as six weeks. The intestinal wall of puppies is highly permeable at this age. Since puppies are commonly switched to a commercial food high in cereal (grain) content, undigested grain protein enters the dog's system early on.

As a contrast, consider again, the wild dog. Pups in the wild still nurse from their mother, on and off, until about three months of age. Until that time, their immature bodies are not able or ready to digest all forms of solid food. This is a very different scenario than that faced by domesticated puppies.

The second example of infiltration may simply be a continuation of the damage begun in puppyhood. Some adult dogs exhibit problems with IgA production. The body either produces *excess* amounts of IgA or *insufficient* amounts of IgA. In cases of excessive IgA production, an overkill effect takes place. The antibodies begin to attack anything around them, including the healthy tissue of the intestine. In cases of insufficient IgA production, antibodies are unable to completely line the intestinal wall. Gaps exist between them. This condition is referred to as **IgA deficiency.**

In either case, large protein molecules, including the protein molecules of grain, are able to pass through these new spaces. In fact, since grain is the major ingredient in commercial foods, it is statistically likely that grain protein crosses the intestinal wall most often.

When infiltration occurs, the body reacts to these large protein molecules as if they are invaders, not food sources. The second line of defense is deployed. **IgG** and **IgM** antibodies infiltrate the area. These antibodies attack and destroy the large protein molecules just as if the protein were a viral infection. **IgE** antibodies cause the release of **histamine**, a natural chemical in the body, which is also designed to fight invaders.

Histamine is responsible for the signs we see in **allergic reactions**. If histamine targets the skin tissue, the result is itchiness, swelling, and rash. If it targets the GI tract, signs can include swelling, irritation, vomiting, and diarrhea. This condition is often referred to as **inflammatory bowel disease**.

Dogs with this condition may exhibit episodes of frantic behavior. They may slobber, lick their lips, or eat household items (such as pillows or carpeting) in an attempt to soothe their irritation. Chronic inflammation of the bowel can impair absorption of prescription medications and important minerals such as magnesium, calcium, and phosphorus. In addition, chronic inflammation allows the liver to absorb the toxic chemicals present in commercial food.

Since IgA also lines the mucous membranes of the lungs and bladder, it is common to find disruptions in those organs, as well. These may include urinary tract infections, calcium deposits, pulmonary edema (fluid in the lungs), and thromboemboli (blood clots).

The immune system responds to inflammation by releasing more **cortisol**, the steroid/hormone produced by the adrenal glands. Cortisol attempts to reduce the bowel inflammation. Unfortunately, the long-term presence of excess cortisol can have myriad negative effects elsewhere in the body. These dogs may begin to exhibit the signs of **Cushing's disease**.

To review, a second hormone called adrenocorticotrophic hormone (ACTH) controls the secretion of cortisol. A feedback loop exists within the body to keep these powerful hormones in balance. When the body is stressed, ACTH is released into the bloodstream. This produces an even greater demand upon the adrenal glands to secrete cortisol.

Because the levels of ACTH and cortisol are constantly fluctuating, they may periodically fall within normal levels. Bloodwork done at these times may suggest that the dog is normal, when indeed, those findings are actually false. This is one reason a dog may test false for the disease while exhibiting significant signs of excess cortisol.

In healthy dogs, the body recognizes that sufficient levels of cortisol are present, and curtails the release of ACTH. This, in turn, stops cortisol production. Normally it is a finely tuned system. However, if inflammation persists over time, the adrenal glands wear out from sustained effort. Ultimately, some dogs may produce insufficient levels of cortisol or cortisol that is weak and **biologically inactive**.

When cortisol levels are too high or too low, they can have a detrimental effect on the immune system. Excess levels of cortisol (or synthetic cortisone/prednisone) depress the immune system, and initially hamper the production of antibodies. Low levels or inactive cortisol exert insufficient control over the immune system, causing antibody production to go a bit haywire. Biologically inactive cortisol interferes with the activity of white blood cells and the production of antibodies. Either scenario can contribute to faulty IgA production.

Furthermore, biologically inactive cortisol does not register with the pituitary gland as "real" cortisol. The feedback loop to the pituitary gland is never shut off. The pituitary gland continues to secrete ACTH in a misguided attempt to raise cortisol levels. These dogs have high levels of ACTH and cortisol circulating in their bloodstream. This can skew the results of dexamethasone tests, causing doctors difficulty as they attempt to differentiate between adrenal tumors and pituitary-dependent Cushing's.

It is well-accepted in human medicine that when an organ is required to function excessively it becomes hypertrophied and exhausted. Degeneration usually follows. Add to this scenario a depressed immune system, a genetic predisposition, and known carcinogens in the diet, and you may have the perfect recipe for a tumor of the pituitary or adrenal glands.

Exhausted adrenal glands may no longer be able to respond to stress and may result in a false negative ACTH test. Adrenal exhaustion also causes magnesium to be lost from the body, as reflected by an increase in urinary output. This can result in a vicious cycle, since magnesium is required as a basic building block to manufacture hormones.

ACTH also stimulates the adrenal glands to produce estrogen (This is different from the *ovarian* estrogen necessary for pregnancy. **Adrenal estrogen** is involved in immune system function and closely resembles cortisol.) Excess estrogen also suppresses the activity of the white blood cells and antibodies. This may be another contributing factor to faulty IgA production.

Estrogen binds with, and inactivates, several hormones. The first of these is **thyroid hormone**, which regulates the body's metabolic rate. (This is a separate phenomenon from the most common cause of hypothyroidism — autoimmune disease.) Certain thyroid tests performed on these dogs may identify normal *levels* of thyroid, but such tests do not recognize that the hormone has been rendered inactive. Inactive or insufficient levels of thyroid hormone slow metabolism. Estrogen also binds with, and inactivates, what little active cortisol *is* present. This can continue the vicious cycle of ACTH production.

When the immune system is healthy, white blood cells are able to distinguish between friend (food molecule) and foe (invaders). But when the immune system is highly stressed, as in the scenario described here, it fails to make this distinction. This is when the serious trouble begins.

Antibodies that have been previously programmed to attack a foreign amino acid chain *recognize that same chain* somewhere else in the dog's own body. The immune system can no longer make the distinction between self and non-self. Antibodies attack healthy tissue.

If the immune system attacks the thyroid gland, the result is lymphocytic thyroiditis or hypothyroidism. If the body attacks the red blood cells, the result is autoimmune hemolytic anemia. In the case of diabetes mellitus, the antibodies recognize a similar protein chain in the pancreas. They destroy the beta cells and their ability to produce insulin. The connection between IgA deficiency, grain protein, and autoimmune disease is so well accepted in human healthcare that it has a nickname. It is called the "leaky gut syndrome."

Fats in Commercial Foods

Dietary fat is blamed for a host of problems in dogs, including pancreatitis. This idea warrants closer examination. Dogs *do* require a certain amount of fat in their diet, so it should not be considered as the all-evil ingredient. In fact, contemporary literature suggests that dogs utilize dietary fat as a primary source of energy — fat that is of high *quality*.

Fats, like protein, used in commercial dog food are usually very poor quality. They can consist of restaurant grease, often rancid and deemed unfit-for-humans, or the tallow that rises from vats of 4-D meats at rendering plants. Poor quality fat is responsible for the particular (rarely pleasant) odor of pet food. It is sprayed on to most commercial kibble to entice a dog to eat it.

Consider again that puppies cannot digest all solid food early on. A fair comparison might be how we slowly and carefully offer solid food to our own children. We do not sit them down to a holiday dinner in their infancy.

The type of fat in most commercial foods (rancid and heavily preserved) is especially difficult for puppies to digest. It is devoid of its natural enzyme, lipase. Without sufficient lipase, the pancreas must work very hard to digest it. This places one of the earliest stresses on the dog's pancreas.

Poor quality fat irritates a puppy's sensitive intestinal lining. This leads to destruction of the epithelial cells and permanent, life-long scarring of the intestinal wall. This can cause the dog difficulty in recycling bile salts later in life. When the body is unable to reabsorb bile, it accumulates in the small intestine. Dogs often rid themselves of accumulated bile by regurgitating it. Usually this occurs in the early hours of the morning, when the dog's stomach is empty.

Intestinal scarring causes absorption problems. When absorption problems exist, undigested dietary fat is allowed to pass into the large intestine. The normal bacteria present in the large intestine convert the dietary fat to ricinoleic acid. This is the major ingredient in castor oil and a highly effective laxative. The result is diarrhea. Since nutrients such as vitamins A, D, and E are fat soluble (transported into the body only via lipids) disruptions in bile recycling and intestinal scarring inhibit the absorption of these vitamins, as well.

Finally, in cases where the immune system is responding to dietary irritants and invaders, the lymph system is heavily engaged in the production of white blood cells. As a result, the absorption of fatty acids (usually handled by the lymph system) is interrupted. This also contributes to poor digestion of dietary lipids.

Summary

Consider the rather vicious cycle we have just discussed: Puppies experience initial intestinal scarring and protein infiltration when weaned on to commercial food at an early age.

Intestinal scarring interferes with the re-absorption of bile salts.

Eating a lifetime diet of processed food places a great demand on the pancreas to produce digestive enzymes.

Unable to keep up with demand, the pancreas becomes enlarged and inflamed.

White blood cells bring additional enzymes to supplement digestion, neglecting their job to protect the body from invaders.

Digestion is slowed.

Slowed digestion allows ample time for harsh chemicals and foreign molecules to irritate the pancreas, liver and intestinal lining.

The irritation and otherwise-occupied white blood cells provide continued opportunities for large grain protein or other foreign molecules to infiltrate the intestine.

Constant inflammation of the pancreas, liver, and intestinal lining results in a sustained production of cortisol.

The adrenal glands, exhausted from this sustained effort, may produce cortisol that is biologically inactive.

Biologically inactive cortisol fails to shut off the ACTH feedback loop. The pituitary gland may become hypertrophied and exhausted.

Excessive cortisol production, prescription steroids, intestinal scarring, and the otherwise-occupied white blood cells hamper IgA production.

IgA deficiency allows for the continued infiltration of large protein molecules into the body.

IgG and IgM antibodies are deployed, which memorize the amino acid chains of the large protein molecules, and attempt to destroy them.

IgG and IgM antibodies later recognize that same amino acid chain elsewhere in the dog's own body. Unable to distinguish between self and non-self, the antibodies destroy these tissues, as well.

And a lymphatic system preoccupied with immune function (the production of more white blood cells) interferes with lipid digestion.

The whole situation seems a bit like the chicken-and-the-egg puzzle. Dog owners want to know which of their dog's health problems initiated the others. In reality, these conditions are not *precipitated* by one another, at all. These problems are simply different expressions of the *same root problem* — commercial pet food. The results include: digestive problems, immune system problems, and problems of excess cortisol production, or "the threefold effect."

Many dogs today exhibit some degree of endocrine/digestive/immune disease. They suffer from skin infections, allergies, autoimmune disorders, vomiting, diarrhea, obesity, hypothyroidism, urinary tract infections, and incontinence. *Which particular* disorder they develop is likely a matter of genetic predisposition, but clearly, many of our pets are experiencing the same underlying problem.

Think of metabolic disease as a continuum. It develops over time and follows a gradual progression. During this time, the body repeatedly substitutes one metabolic function for another. Depending upon where a dog falls along the high-cortisol continuum, he may or may not actually test positive for specific conditions like Cushing's disease. In some respects this is a credit to how well the body can continually adapt to physiological stress.

Notice how closely the factors that contribute to diabetes are related to those that contribute to Cushing's disease, *and* pancreatitis, *and* bowel disease, *and* liver and kidney dysfunction. They are interrelated. Complications occur simultaneously because the entire endocrine/digestive/immune complex is severely stressed. Since metabolic adaptations can be progress for some time, owners may not realize the severity of the situation until the dog's entire system is taxed. ✳

The threefold effect of commercial pet food:

Problems of Excess Cortisol Production:
calcium stones, tooth loss, cognitive changes,
insomnia, incontinence, heart failure

Digestive Problems:
pancreatitis, malabsorption
of lipids, kidney damage

Immune System Problems:
inflammation, allergies and
autoimmune diseases

**Commercial
Pet Food**

Chapter 8

Dietary Management

To most dog owners, dog food means prepared food purchased commercially. This is a relatively new trend, however. Companion dogs have been eating processed foods for the just the last several decades. This is the same time span in which dogs have experienced an alarming increase in digestive and autoimmune diseases. Few people realize how damaging commercial pet food can be.

A Review of Commercial Diets

As early as 1979, *Consumers Digest* questioned the logic of feeding highly processed, grain-based diets to pets. They reported, "There is mounting evidence that a lifetime of eating commercial pet foods can shorten your pet's life, make him fatter than he ought to be, and contribute to the development of such increasingly common disorders as cystitis and stones (in cats), glaucoma and heart disease (in dogs), diabetes, lead poisoning, rickets, and serious vitamin-mineral deficiencies (in both cats and dogs)."

All that being said, many dog owners will still choose to feed their dogs commercial diets. Perhaps this is due to the convenience commercial foods offer, owners' doubt about challenging a veterinarian's advice and trying something new, or the very effective advertising campaigns of the pet food industry.

The following guidelines are recommended for dog owners who choose to feed their dogs commercial diets: avoid foods preserved with BHT, BTA, or ethoxyquin. Seek foods that have high quality, human-grade ingredients. Seek foods that do not have rendered fats. And seek foods with the lowest levels of grain products.

These types of food are most often found through holistic veterinarians, holistic pet supply shops, or over the Internet. In addition, consider supplementing commercial diets with some fresh foods, or digestive enzymes. (See the Suppliers section or contact your veterinarian.)

Hints for Finicky Eaters

The final problem with commercial foods (particularly the "diet" and prescription formulations) is that they are unpalatable. Many dogs don't like them. This becomes a crucial issue, since diabetic dogs must eat when receiving insulin injections. Refusal to eat can precipitate a hypoglycemic episode and a potentially deadly situation.

There are several other issues that may cause a dog to lose interest in food. Diabetic and Cushinoid dogs are frequently placed on antibiotic therapy for various infections. Antibiotics often cause GI upset. Discomfort from pancreatitis is another common cause of appetite loss in dogs. Individual diabetic dogs may experience loss of appetite when blood glucose levels are very high *or* very low.

Dog owners have devised some clever ways to make meals more appealing to their pets. Some dog owners spread a spoonful of canned cat food or tuna fish on top of the kibble. Others have had success with low-sodium, low-fat chicken broth or canned (jars of) baby food meats. Look for baby foods that do not list sugar on the label. Other owners have had success adding small amounts of Parmesan cheese, cottage cheese, or yogurt. Discuss your intentions with your veterinarian.

In cases where dogs refuse to eat, you may be instructed to force feed a meal. This can be accomplished by placing canned food or a homemade meal into the blender with enough water to create a thick liquid. This solution can be poured into a large syringe or turkey baster and inserted at the side of the dog's mouth. Try not to aim for the back of the mouth as this may cause the dog to choke. You may only be able to inject a small amount at a time. Talk to your dog reassuringly during and after the procedure.

Another option is to prepare the mixture with less water and include a sticky ingredient such as canned pumpkin (not pie filling) or banana. You may be able to wipe small fingerful amounts on the dog's upper palate. Some food will be wasted but some will be ingested. Many pets, even when uninterested in other food, will drink the water in which tuna fish is packed. This can be helpful when dehydration is a concern.

More Wholesome Options for Feeding

At this point, some readers may wish to abandon the practice of feeding commercial foods. They may have feelings of guilt or even anger regarding the misinformation they've been given in the past. This is normal. Remember that as pet owners, we do the best we can with the information we have. The pet-food industry continues to teach consumers that dogs are only supposed to eat what comes out of a bag or a can.

Diets Prepared at Home

It is ludicrous to debate whether dogs can be maintained in good health on homemade diets. In the thousands of years since humans and dogs first began their friendship, humans have shared the food from their own hunt/farm/dining table with their dogs. It has only been in the last several decades that commercial food has been available for pets. This represents an abrupt change from a diet that has lasted for centuries.

Some people are direly afraid that they will not be able to get canine nutrition "right" for their pet. The pet food industry has convinced them that the practice of dog feeding is a complex science and that every meal must be completely and painstakingly balanced according to dubious industry standards. The concept of creating carbon-copy meals is highly artificial and even detrimental. Humans and dogs alike were designed to achieve a balanced diet *over time*. We were never designed to eat the same meals every day of our entire lives.

If commercial diets truly offered the excellent nutrition they advertise, dog owners would not be supplementing these foods with a never-ending parade of vitamins, minerals, herbs, and oils. Rather than discussing the practice of supplementing poor quality commercial foods, this text will instead examine the value of switching to a home-prepared diet. If you can feed yourself and your family, you can feed your dog, too.

Preparing a Home-cooked Diet

Pet owners frequently express uncertainty when switching to a home-cooked diet. They want to have hard, fast rules to follow. Feeding a chronically ill dog rarely follows strict rules, however. Here are some guidelines to follow, but you and your veterinarian will still need to discuss your dog's ongoing condition, weight, and metabolism.

The *most current* recommendation for preparing a cooked diet at home is as follows:

The diet should consist of approximately 50% meat (ground meat such as beef, turkey, or chicken); organ meat, eggs, and fish, such as sardines; as well as the occasional *cultured* milk product, such as plain yogurt or kefir.

If you chose to add grain to your dog's diet, feed no more than about one-sixth of the diet, or 15%, as grain.

The remainder, 35% to 50% should consist of vegetables and fruits, preferably pulped or blended in a food processor.

Feeding Dogs With Kidney Disease or Pancreatitis

This diet is easily adapted to dogs with special needs. If your dog suffers from pancreatitis, use lean cuts of meat. Drain away any cooked fat and grease from the meat. Remember that commercial dog food damages the GI tract early in puppyhood. This makes fat digestion difficult, if not nearly impossible for some dogs. Consider adding digestive enzymes to the diet. Feeding small, frequent meals may also be helpful as it places less stress on the pancreas.

Dogs suffering from kidney disease may benefit from reduced levels of protein (30% to 40%) and increased levels of the vegetable mixture (60% to 70%.) High quality protein and the comparative lack of chemicals in homemade diets will also ease the strain on kidney function. Avoid foods high in phosphorus and potassium. (See page 60.)

Meal preparation may seem awkward at first, but as with any habit, it becomes faster and easier with time. Most dog owners feeding home-cooked meals basically prepare a stew. Some cook the meat in a skillet, a Dutch oven/crock pot, or microwave oven. If they choose to feed grains, they cook or soak them beforehand, then add them to the meat. Vegetables are finely chopped or pulped and then added to the mixture. Other owners mix together ground meat and chopped vegetables and cook, resulting in the equivalent of a doggy-meatloaf.

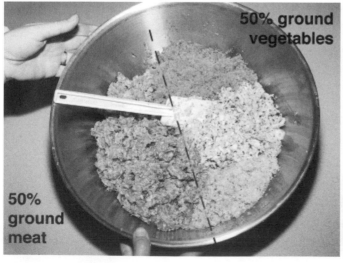

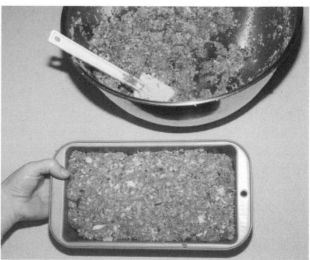

If you are dealing with diseases other than diabetes, it is possible to take an even more relaxed approach to feeding. Some owners feed a variety of foods that they themselves are eating. This may include such items as pasta with meat and tomato sauce; leftover meats such as cooked fish, roast beef, chicken (with *cooked* bones removed); leftover baked potatoes, vegetables, and over-ripe fruit. When leftovers are scarce, they may bake a potato and top it with a can of tuna or sardines, or a soft-boiled egg or two.

Eggs are an excellent addition to the diet. The protein in eggs is easily digested and has a high degree of bioavailability. And eggs contain **lecithin**, a nutrient that helps emulsify dietary fat and lower cholesterol. Sardines contain omega fatty acids which are thought to have anitinflammatory properties.

Many veterinarians and pet food company salesmen will frown upon this approach, and yet, it is the way in which dogs have been successfully fed for decades. Owners may notice one other important benefit of feeding this way. They may begin eating better themselves. Many people notice an improvement in their own health when they replace highly processed, heavily preserved foods with those that are whole and fresh.

Above and beyond this basic formulation (50% meat, 35% to 50% vegetables, and no more than 15% grain) there are some fine points you may wish to consider. When cooking meats, cook them lightly (rare or medium-rare). Meats cooked well-done are devoid of intrinsic enzymes. Meats can include ground meat or larger cuts, as well as organ meats such as liver, kidneys, and heart. *Always* cook salmon for dogs and remove any cooked bones.

If you choose to add grain to your dog's diet, consider oatmeal. Oatmeal seems to be one of the least offending grains to dogs. Owners of diabetic dogs also find it to be an effective way to add fiber to the diet. Oatmeal can be cooked, or soaked overnight in water or yogurt.

Other excellent sources of fiber include pumpkin (plain, not "pie-filling" which contains sugar). Pumpkin also helps **control diarrhea**. Celery, apples and broccoli, stems and all, are other good sources of fiber. Some owners even add a spoonful of Metamucil to the diet. Based on a biologically appropriate approach, large amounts of grains and bran products should be avoided. Fiber is best supplied from fruit and vegetable sources.

It is strongly recommended that you pulp fruits and vegetables in a blender or food processor. Dogs have difficulty breaking down the cell walls of plant material. When you break foods down mechanically, the dog's digestive system has better access to the nutrients. In addition, *do* cook such vegetables as potatoes, yams and squash. Other vegetables can be served *either* cooked or raw.

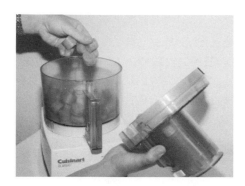 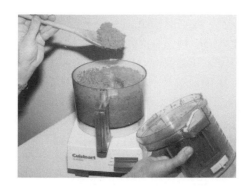

The following vegetables are considered rather **high in sugar** and should be fed sparingly to dogs with unregulated DM, skin allergies or obesity: potatoes, carrots, winter squash, and green peas. *Low sugar* vegetables include dark leafy greens such as spinach and lettuce, kale, celery, cabbage, and broccoli. These are also good sources of **vitamin E**, which may support visual function. Dark, leafy vegetables are also high in **magnesium**, as are apples, sunflower seeds, nuts, bananas, parsley, peanut butter, meat and fish. Sufficient levels of magnesium may help reduce signs of weakness, irritability, hair loss, insulin resistance and the formation of calcium based kidney stones.

Foods such as corn, yogurt, tomatoes, beans, peas, nuts, oatmeal, sardines, bran, spinach, sweet potatoes, cheese and bananas are **high in potassium** content. Meat, yeast, grain, canned fish, nuts, eggs, and potatoes are **high in phosphorus**. Avoid or reduce the latter in cases of kidney degeneration.

Healthy dogs eating *cooked* diets should receive some calcium and phosphorus supplementation. If your dog suffers from alterations in calcium metabolism (see page 24), consider adding magnesium to the diet. This may help lower serum calcium levels by moving calcium back into bone and cartilidge.

If you do add calcium and phosphorus to the diet, be advised that a certain amount of debate exists as to the best source of these minerals. Some dog owners add 1/2 teaspoon of ground eggshells for every pound of meat. They save their eggshells, grind them in a coffee grinder and store them in the refrigerator until needed. Some use bone meal. Others use prepared vitamin/mineral supplements available from pet supply shops and veterinarians. Also, consider supplementing fully cooked diets with digestive enzymes. This will help ease the workload on the pancreas.

Dog owners frequently ask, "How *much* food should I give my dog?" One rule of thumb recommends that a dog's daily food intake should equal 2% to 3% of his body-weight. Dogs are individuals, though. They have different metabolic rates. Some dogs are "high energy" individuals requiring more calories, and others are not. The overall state of the dog's immune system will have an effect on his metabolic rate, too. What this means is that dietary recommendations are simply suggestions, and you may have to adjust the levels of ingredients as your dog's metabolism stabilizes.

If your dog is diabetic, settle on a formulation that agrees with both of you, and measure out uniform amounts of ingredients for each new batch of stew. This will provide the same consistency (if not more) than commercial food provides and some veterinarians insist upon. Some owners who test their dog's blood glucose levels at home (see page 105), vary the ingredients, supplying a healthy variety of nutrients. This concept also applies to feeding dogs with pancreatitis and Cushing's disease. This is the way in which dogs (and people) were naturally designed to eat.

You can save yourself time and energy by making enough stew for about a week's worth of meals. Divide the stew into freezer-bag portions or small containers and freeze them. You will quickly get in the habit of taking out one bag to defrost whenever you feed your dog.

The Benefits of Feeding Home-cooked Diets

The benefits of feeding your dog a home-cooked meal are numerous. Your dog will be ingesting few, if any, preservatives, chemicals, or dyes. He will be receiving ingredients of *much* higher quality and nutritional value. And you can virtually eliminate grains from the diet.

Homemade diets also appear to reduce the need for insulin, which can be an economic consideration. They can and do reduce clinical signs such as polydipsia, polyuria, skin infections, diarrhea, lethargy, and muscle weakness. Dog owners have even reported forestalling previously imminent increases in Cushing's medications after switching their dogs to homemade diets.

Home-cooked meals are immensely palatable to dogs. If your dog has been finicky in the past, he is much more likely to now eat reliably. Home-cooked meals can be prepared with as much consistency of ingredients as any commercial foods. Finally, dog-owners frequently describe a feeling of satisfaction from making their dogs a real meal.

Will a homemade diet *cure* diabetes, Cushing's disease, pancreatitis, kidney or liver failure? Probably not, as damage done early in life may still result in health problems. However, a more wholesome, appropriate diet *is* likely to aid immune system function, reduce inflammation and clinical symptoms, improve quality of life, and add to a dog's longevity.

The Drawbacks of Feeding Home-cooked Diets

Preparing homemade dog food may also have some drawbacks for your family. It will require more of your time. It will require more of your freezer space.

And it is likely to cost you about the same or more than premium or prescription dog foods. Offset costs by purchasing ingredients at warehouse-style grocery stores or by asking the butcher to order you dog's meat in bulk.

It is also possible for home-cooked diets to have some of the same drawbacks as commercial diets. If you cook food at high temperatures, amino acids, enzymes, and some vitamins will be damaged. If you choose to feed large amounts of grain, your dog may experience many of the same immune system problems he has from eating a commercial diet.

While the concept of preparing a "stew" provides consistency in the diabetic's diet, it too has drawbacks. When all the food elements (proteins, carbohydrates, fats, and minerals) are present at the same meal, some of them combine in unfortunate ways. Proteins and certain minerals can form "complexes" with carbohydrates and various lipids, rendering them unavailable.

And yet, even the most over-cooked, stew-styled, home-prepared meal is an incredible improvement over commercial dog food. Additionally, the argument still remains that for many, many years, dogs have been living long healthy lives while sharing his owner's cooked table scraps.

Raw Food Diets

Dog owners have another option in preparing meals at home. This is the Biologically Appropriate Raw Food diet, also known as the Bones and Raw Food diet, or BARF. This diet attempts (within limits) to reproduce the diet of the wolf and wild dog. It consists of raw meat or raw meaty bones (such as chicken necks, wings, and backs) and mostly raw fruits and vegetables.

Many pet owners are now convinced that this type of nutrition is necessary for their pets to achieve optimum health. In the 1940s, Dr. Francis Pottinger Jr. did a series of controlled studies that supports this belief. His studies demonstrated that cats fed raw diets were far more healthy and resistant to disease and developmental abnormalities than cats fed the same cooked foods. Even so, the BARF diet is poorly accepted by the traditional veterinary community. The two most commonly cited objections are fear of feeding bones and fear of bacteria.

Remember the natural design of the dog. The teeth are designed to tear meat and crunch bones. Wild dogs routinely consume the bones of their prey as part of their meal. As Dr. Ian Billinghurst points out in his book "Give Your Dog a Bone," it is *cooked bones*, not raw bones, that cause dogs problems such as GI perforations. *Cooked bones* shatter and splinter. Raw bones are soft and digested by the dog's strong stomach acids.

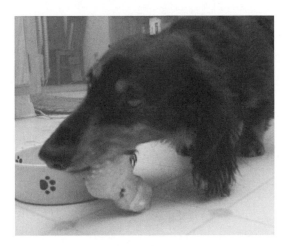 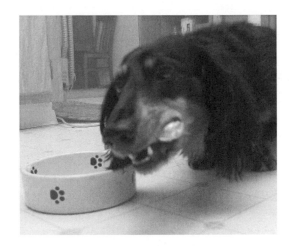

In years past, owners commonly gave their pets raw meaty bones from their own farms, ranches, or butchers. Pet food companies, and their strong influence in veterinary schools, have steered owners away from this practice. The omission of meaty bones from the canine diet has paralleled the development of veterinary dentistry. Dogs that chewed raw bones had clean teeth naturally. They did not require dental chew toys, toothbrushes, or surgical procedures with general anesthesia to maintain normal dental health.

Many people have been taught to have an undue fear of germs. The reality is that dogs regularly come into contact with bacteria, including e-coli and salmonella, on a daily basis. Such contact is an integral part of canine behavior. It is normal for these bacteria to be present in the canine digestive tract.

Given the chance, many dogs will roll in the droppings and carcasses of other animals. Dogs will eat these things, too. They will bury chew toys in dirt, and contentedly gnaw on them later. Most common of all, dogs groom their own hind ends! Dogs come in contact with these "dangerous" bacteria all day long. Their bodies were designed to handle them. In fact, it is *important* that dogs come in contact with germs so that they develop immunity. Only dogs with weakened immune systems or prolonged antibiotic use face a threat from bacterial overgrowth.

Another argument you may hear opposing raw food is that "just because wolves eat a certain way, doesn't mean pet dogs should, too. After all, wild dogs die much younger than our pets do." This argument is not valid. The Grey Wolf lives an average of 10 to 12 years in the wild. Most of us know of at least one dog that died prematurely, either from cancer or other serious illness. Of the domestic dogs that *do* live longer, many are subjected to chronic, expensive, painful diseases in ever-increasing numbers.

That being said, it is important to introduce raw foods to chronically ill dogs, *slowly*. Their immune systems are already compromised. Their pancreatic function is taxed. Their organs are inflamed. These dogs will need help in assimilating the rich supply of nutrients a fresh diet can provide.

Preparing a Raw Food Diet

There are two basic methods of preparing a BARF diet. Neither one includes much, if any, grain product. In the first method, meat meals are served separately from vegetable meals. This separation prevents various nutrients from binding together, which can render them unavailable. It also provides the kidneys with a much-needed rest. Meals consisting mainly of vegetables put little demand on kidney function.

About 50% to 70% of the diet should consist of raw meaty bones (RMBs.) This can include chicken necks, wings, or backs. RMBs are different than large joint bones. RMBs are crunched up by the dog and consumed as meals. They contain a biologically appropriate ratio of meat, calcium, and phosphorus. You may wish to remove the excess fat and skin if your dog suffers from pancreatitis or obesity. Running warm water over RMBs will help bring them to room temperature before serving.

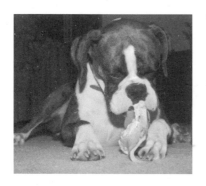

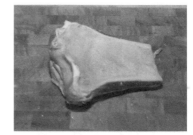

Joint bones (also called knuckle or soup bones) also have a place in the BARF diet. They provide an excellent way to entertain both overly energetic and lethargic dogs. Joint bones, too, should be offered raw, as cooked bones can break into dangerous shards. Throw bones away when they get small as some overly ambitious dogs might try to swallow them whole.

The second version of the raw food diet offers meat and vegetables together. This mimics the basic "stew" concept discussed previously, which does have advantages in regulating diabetic dogs. In this method RMBs may either be offered intact or passed through a meat grinding machine. This appeals to those dog owners who simply cannot accept the idea of feeding whole bones. (See Suppliers Section for commercial meat grinders.)

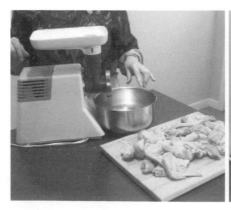
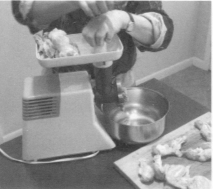
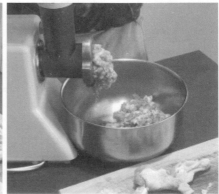

With either method, diabetic-dog owners might find it helpful to practice glucose testing at home. People who feed raw meals explain that it is easy to adjust ingredients when glucose readings are a bit high or low. Also, home testing allows the dog owner more freedom to include a *variety* of meats and vegetables. It reduces the need for strict consistency from one batch of food to another and it provides the dog with a healthier spectrum of nutrients. This is the way human diabetics manage their own meals.

Vegetable meals can actually contain a variety of things in addition to just vegetables. This includes fruit, organ meat (liver, kidney, heart), eggs, sardines, and yogurt. As previously discussed in the cooked-diet section, vegetables should be finely ground. Starchy vegetables such as potatoes, yams, and squash are actually best cooked.

If you do feed grain, cook it thoroughly or soak it overnight in warm water or yogurt. Some people feed eggs whole and raw, some soft boil them, some cook them fully. The main concern is that raw egg whites contain avidin, which in very large amounts binds with biotin, an essential B vitamin, rendering it unavailable to the body.

If you find that your dog does not enjoy his vegetable meals, try adding a small amount of garlic, tomato sauce, banana, pumpkin, or ground meat (especially liver) in the mixture. Some dog owners add as much as 50% ground meat (muscle meat or organ meat) to the vegetable mixture. Most dogs find these ingredients highly palatable.

Do *not* add calcium supplements to BARF diets. The raw meaty bones will supply appropriate levels of calcium and other minerals. Added supplements may actually cause joint and skeletal problems.

As with cooked diets, it is possible to prepare meals as your schedule permits, and freeze the excess. You will quickly get into the habit of defrosting one container each time you feed your dog. Freezing fresh food does not damage intrinsic enzymes, but may damage the water-soluble vitamins (A and B vitamins) to some degree.

The Benefits of Feeding Raw Food Diets

Feeding your dog fresh, raw foods will supply him with undamaged amino acids, vitamins, minerals, and enzymes. Raw calories are nonstimulating to the pituitary gland and the appetite center in the brain. This helps reduce symptoms of hunger. It helps stabilize body weight. Of all the dietary options, dog owners report the lowest need for insulin when their dogs are eating fresh, raw foods, without grains. The reduction in insulin can be as much as 40% to 50%.

Preparing raw food meals typically takes less time than making home cooked meals (since no cooking is required). They are also more economical since the meaty bones (chicken necks, wings, and backs) are less costly than ground meat or fillets.

Fresh foods contain intact enzymes, greatly reducing stress on the exocrine pancreas. Dogs process this food quickly. Less energy is engaged in digestion and can be diverted to other activities such as immune system function. Biologically appropriate foods are less irritating to the intestinal tract. They place much less stress on kidney and liver function as well.

The Drawbacks of Feeding Raw Food Diets

As with the any diet, the BARF diet does have its drawbacks. It is more time consuming than feeding commercial diets. It requires as much, or more, freezer space as home-cooked diets. If you board your dog at a kennel, or hire a dog-sitter, others may be uncomfortable or unwilling to feed raw food. In these cases, it may be best to provide containers of cooked food for the time you'll be away. And finally, your veterinarian may not be supportive of this concept.

Variations in Homemade Diets

Several variations are possible in the preparation of homemade diets. Some dog owners choose to cook all the ingredients in the diet. Some cook the meat and the grain, leaving the vegetables fresh; others choose to cook the meat only very lightly. Variations also exist in raw food diets. Some owners do not feed bones, until cortisol (and calcium) levels are brought under control. (See page 24.) Dogs without calcium problems may be fed calcium supplements.

Switching Diets

Whether you are switching your dog from one commercial diet to another, or from commercial to homemade, two things apply. It should be done gradually, and it should be done with your veterinarian's knowledge. Make the switch over many weeks. Some individuals may take months. These dogs are likely to have irritated organs throughout their bodies.

The change to a new diet can drastically reduce the amount of insulin needed, as much as 50% in some cases. This is especially true if you are adding fresh foods to your dog's diet. It can also affect the way his body uses nutrients and stores fat. Monitor weight gain and weight loss. Adjust insulin doses and meal size accordingly. Keep your veterinarian apprised of your plans and progress.

To switch from one commercial diet to another commercial diet, exchange a few of the regular kibble for the new kibble, or a spoonful of the regular canned food for the new canned food. Each day add a bit more of the new food and less of the old food. This process should be accomplished slowly, over the course of several weeks.

To switch from a commercial diet to any type of homemade diet, progress especially slowly. Remember that yours is a dog with a compromised immune system and irritated GI tract. Dogs living on commercial diets for long periods may have many inflamed internal organs and absorption problems. They may require extra help in digesting new foods.

Even if you are adding fresh (raw) food that will contain intrinsic enzymes, strongly consider adding digestive enzymes to this diet as your dog first adjusts. These are available at pet supply shops (see Suppliers list) or through veterinarians. It may be possible to eliminate the extra enzymes if a dog's pancreatic function improves. Dietary enzymes may help in the metabolism of fat-soluble vitamins, as well.

Begin the switch by adding meat first (whichever you decide, raw or cooked.) Add small amounts until a ratio of 50% meat to 50% commercial food is reached. Then add the vegetable/mix, a spoonful at a time. Following that step, add any grain products, *if* you choose to do so. As you increase the volume of homemade food, decrease the volume of commercial food.

To switch a dog to the BARF diet, introduce raw meaty bones (chicken necks, wings, or backs) separately from kibble meals. Kibble and raw meaty bones digest quite differently and it is recommended that they not be fed at the same time. Gradually replace 50% to 70% of the kibble meals with RMB meals. Then introduce ground veggie/organ meat/egg, etc. meals to make up the remainder.

Snacks, Treats, and How to Hide Medications

Just because your dog is diabetic, it does not mean an end to snacks and food treats. Snacks are an important element in maintaining a more consistent level of blood sugar during the day. Treats are highly valuable in training dogs to take pills, and to accept insulin injections and blood tests.

If you are feeding a commercial diet, seek out treats that have the lowest levels of grain and highest levels of meat. Avoid treats containing high levels of corn (some synthetic chew bones), rice (rice cakes), and soy (tofu). As previously discussed, dogs are not designed to assimilate these ingredients. Avoid commercial biscuits and treats that have high levels of sugar. Sugar can be listed in any of the following ways: corn syrup, dextrose, glucose, and maltose. Some dog owners have experimented with making "cookies" from canned food. They slice the food and baked it at low temperatures for about thirty minutes.

If you are feeding a homemade diet, you can use a variety of real foods as snacks. Many dogs are fond of raw carrots, bananas, or apples. By some estimates these may be considered high-sugar foods, but it is important to remember that raw sugar and starch are not assimilated the same way they are when cooked. Raw foods do not raise blood sugar levels as much as cooked foods do.

Other owners offer small amounts of protein, such as a slice of roast beef or turkey deli meat. Some owners even prepare homemade meat jerky. This can be made from beef or boneless chicken breasts sliced thinly. Low-sodium soy sauce or garlic powder can be added for extra flavor. The meat is placed in a dehydrator or oven set at 145 degrees F. overnight or for most of the day.

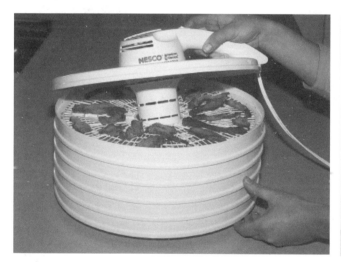
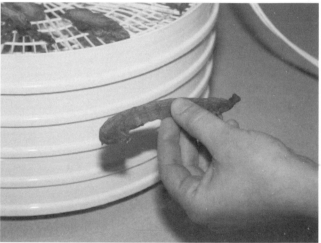

Oral medications or supplements can be hidden inside folded pieces of low-fat luncheon meat. If your dog has transitioned to a raw food diet, you may find chicken hearts to be an excellent vehicle for dispensing pills. (They have a perfect pill-sized cavity.) For very finicky eaters, try cream cheese, liverwurst, or tuna fish. While some of these are higher in fat content, they may help get medication down in worst-case scenarios.

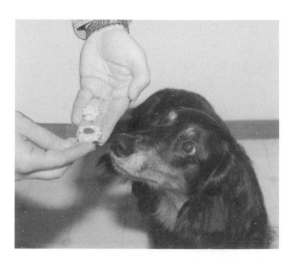

Regardless of the food treat, the "rapid-fire method" is very successful way to medicate dogs. This involves feeding a food treat (with the pill hidden inside) and *immediately* offering a second food treat (without a pill).

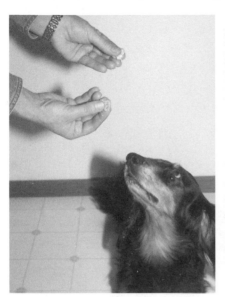 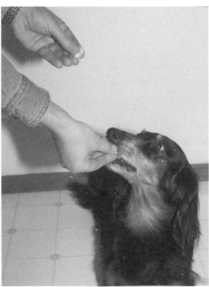 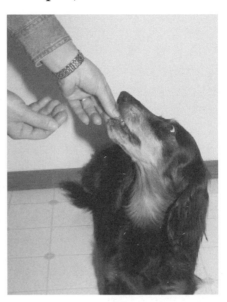

Dogs are usually so interested in getting the second treat, that they readily swallow the first one without taking time to sort out the medication. Build the trust of finicky eaters by offering them a plain treat *prior* to the medicated treat.

Until glucose levels or Cushing's signs become regulated by medications, dogs may exhibit a voracious appetite. This may persist for several months. Excessive snacking can interfere with the process of regulating diabetics because more food requires more insulin. For voracious eaters, try offering low calorie, high fiber snacks such as carrots, celery, or raw beef knuckle bones. They will help distract your dog and fill his stomach for a while.

Water Consumption

It is crucial to provide diabetic and Cushinoid dogs with ample water. Many dog owners are tempted to restrict a dog's water consumption to reduce urinary accidents, but this can have dire consequences. Limiting water intake does *not* reduce urination. Instead, it may result in dehydration. This is a serious situation that can lead to death.

These dogs need access to unlimited water. Check the water bowl frequently. Once a dog becomes regulated, the excessive thirst and urination will subside. Continue to supply ample fresh water, as fluctuations in blood glucose and cortisol levels can cause bouts of thirst, even once regulated.

Changes in Body Weight

Changes in body weight are common as various diseases are brought under control. Diabetic dogs that have lost weight over this time begin to regain it. Weight gain can typically take between three and six months.

If your dog is obese, weight loss should be achieved slowly over a period of several months. Reducing fats and grains in the diet and introducing fresh foods should contribute to weight loss. Monitor your dog's weight on an ongoing basis. (Veterinary clinics usually do not mind if you bring your dog in simply for the purpose of weighing him.) Keep your veterinarian apprised of weight loss. As your dog loses weight, he is likely to require less insulin. This concept is not fully understood, but it is believed that obesity blocks insulin receptor sites.

Other Oral Aids

Dog owners add countless dietary supplements to commercial pet food in an attempt to improve it. To examine the extent of these products is beyond the scope of this book. This author believes that it is healthier to improve the basic diet. All that being said, there are a few oral supplements that may be worthy of your consideration.

Glandular Extracts

Holistic veterinarians sometimes recommend the addition of glandular extracts, or "glandulars" (concentrates of raw animal glands) to the diet. The theory behind glandular extracts is that "cells help like cells." Pancreas, adrenal, and thyroid glandulars are commercially available to the veterinary community, and in some nutritional supplements. (See Suppliers list.)

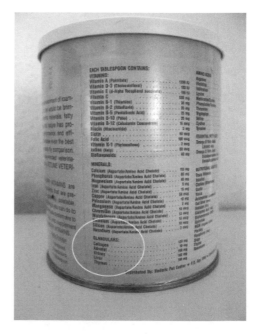

Little scientific data exists on the validity of glandular extracts, but it is interesting to note that studies done at the beginning of the 20th century indicated that human diabetic patients benefited from the oral ingestion of animal pancreas extracts. Eventually, this work led scientists to the discovery and widespread use of injectable insulin, today's most common treatment of Type 1 diabetes.

Melatonin

Veterinary interest is mounting in melatonin, a hormone normally produced in the pineal gland, but also available as an oral supplement. Veterinarians recommend melatonin for a variety of problems including insomnia, neurological and behavioral issues such as epilepsy, aggression, separation anxiety, and fear of loud noises. Melatonin has been used to treat bilateral flank alopecia (hair loss), thyroid disease, obesity, cancer, and immune deficiency disorders.

Phosphatidyl Serine

Some holistic veterinarians also prescribe the oral supplement Phosphatidyl Serine (PS) in cases of excess cortisol production. PS is a natural phospholipid that is normally made by the body through a series of complex processes. Levels deteriorate with age and stress. PS improves nervous system and memory function in humans. Studies also indicate that PS raises circulating levels of such hormones as dopamine and melatonin, and *reduces* levels of ACTH and coritsol.

Phosphatidyl Serine was originally tested on dogs prior to FDA approval for use in humans. Adverse effects were not noted in these dogs after prolonged use on high doses. The average dose for *human* use is 300 mg per day. The owners of small dogs (weighing 10 to 25 pounds) have reported reduced symptoms of cortisol with 50 mg to 100 mg per day. The owner's of medium sized dogs (weighing 40 to 50 pounds) have reported good results with 200 mg per day. Reduced symptoms are often noted in 2 to 3 weeks.

Dietary therapy (including the addition of PS) may be especially helpful in the following two situations:
1) in the absence of a formal Cushing's diagnosis, and
2) when a dog is poorly controlled with traditional Cushing's medications.
 While PS is available at most health food stores and does not require a doctor's prescription, it is still wise to keep your veterinarian apprised of your plans.

Summary

Canine nutrition is an area of considerable controversy, and the veterinary community admits that not all dietary issues are well understood. For a diet to be successful, however, it must make both the animal and owner happy. If you have strong feelings about trying a new diet, it is helpful to find a veterinarian who will support you in this pursuit. You can ask the staff of a prospective veterinary clinic how the doctor feels about home-prepared or raw food diets.

Even though damage to the digestive tract occurs early in a dog's life, the body can patch a failing metabolic system for some time. It can take years for the extent of the damage to become apparent. With the advent of each additional health problem, dog owners may mistakenly conclude that the new, more whole some diet is responsible. Likewise, they may not believe the new diet is helpful if it doesn't improve matters immediately. It can take six months or more to ease the damage caused by a lifetime of eating kibble.

Allow at least a month's time before deciding whether a new diet is working for a diabetic dog. Pets suffering from pancreatitis and inflammatory bowel syndrome may require *many* months to make the transition. Make this time as easy as possible for your dog, using a gradual approach, high quality ingredients, and digestive enzyme supplements.

Since this book is not intended to be an solely a nutrition text, you are encouraged to investigate these suggested reading materials:

Books and Literature About Commercial Pet Foods:

"Foods Pets Die For: Shocking Facts About Pet Food", by Ann N. Martin, New Sage Press

"Pet Food Investigative Report: The Truth About Commercial Pet Food", by the Animal Protection Institute of America, available on the World Wide Web at http://www.api4animals.org/petfood.htm or free of charge by contacting:
Animal Protection Institute of America
PO Box 22505
Sacramento, CA 95822-2831
(916) 731-5521

"The Nature of Animal Healing: The Path to Your Pet's Health, Happiness and Longevity", by Martin Goldstein, DVM, Alfred A Knopf (publisher)

Books About Biologically Appropriate Raw Food Diets:

"Give Your Dog a Bone: The Practical Commonsense Way to Feed Dogs For a Long Healthy Life", by Ian Billinghurst, BVSc. (Hons), BSc.Agr, Dip. Ed., self-published

"The Ultimate Diet: Natural Nutrition for Dogs and Cats", by Kymythy R. Schultz, AHI, Affenbar Ink

✳

Chapter 9

Caring for Dogs With Diabetes Mellitus

Diabetes mellitus is best treated with a multifaceted approach. This means your dog's meals will be regulated to provide a certain measure of consistency and that insulin will be provided (via injection) to transport glucose into the cells. It also means that you will need to monitor your dog's exercise. This will help control obesity and avoid episodes of low blood sugar.

Some owners will opt to keep the treatment plan simple. This approach involves feeding the dog a commercial diet and giving insulin injections at home. The veterinarian may encourage the dog owner to monitor urine glucose levels, but in this approach, only the veterinarian will draw and test the dog's *blood* glucose levels. This will be done at the clinic.

Other dog owners will opt for a more aggressive treatment plan. Besides giving daily insulin injections, these owners may prepare their dog's meals from scratch and monitor blood glucose levels, themselves, at home.

An Overview of Insulin Activity

Insulin is a protein molecule. While the shape and structure of insulin molecules may differ between species (human, canine, bovine, etc.), they function similarly. Specific sites on the insulin molecule bind with receptor sites on each cell wall. (Remember the analogy of the doorman placing his hand on the doorknob.) Once the "door is opened," glucose can leave the bloodstream, cross the cell wall, and provide the cell with nutrition.

Several terms are used to describe the characteristics and activity of an insulin injection. These include onset, peak, nadir, and duration. **Onset** refers to the length of time required for the insulin to be absorbed from the injection site into the bloodstream. Once there, it will *begin* moving glucose out of the bloodstream and into the cells, lowering blood glucose levels. This is considered to be the onset. When the majority of insulin has been absorbed, it will demonstrate its *greatest action*, or **peak** activity. At that time, *blood glucose levels will be also at their lowest.* This is known as the **nadir.** Each injection of insulin works for finite amount of time. **Duration** refers to the *total length of time* the insulin is effective.

Remember that the *peak in insulin activity* results in the *lowest level of blood glucose.* Ask your veterinarian to describe when your dog's insulin peaks (how long after the injection will the blood sugar be lowest) and how long the insulin will last (duration.) As you read further, you will understand why this information is important.

Also note that the following illustrations and graphs are simply examples. They do not necessarily represent ideal or recommended glucose levels.

Insulin types that have a short onset will usually have a sharp and potent peak in action. Those that have a later onset usually demonstrate a smoother peak and longer duration. Other factors that can affect insulin activity include injection technique, insulin quality, and the response of the individual animal. It is possible for insulin activity to vary slightly from day to day.

Types of Insulin

With each passing year, new formulations of insulin are added to the market, just as others are removed. Discussing insulin types by name carries with it the risk of printing outdated material, however an understanding of your dog's particular insulin will be an important factor in treating his diabetes.

To better understand commercial insulin types, it is helpful to sort them into various categories. The two most common ways of categorizing insulin are by activity (onset, duration, etc.) or source.

Insulin categorized by activity:

Insulin activity in pets is generally of a much shorter duration than insulin activity in humans. The time frames discussed here have been estimated for dogs. Individual dogs can have widely varying experiences.

Short-acting insulin usually includes the word regular or the abbreviation R in its name, such as Regular, Novalin R, and Humulin R. Onset of action is rapid, usually less than 30 minutes. It peaks between 1 and 4 hours, and duration is short, between 3 and 8 hours. Short-acting insulin is most often used in emergency cases of ketoacidosis, as it quickly lowers blood glucose levels.

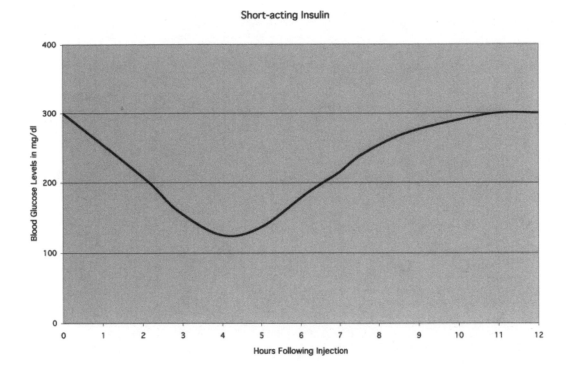

Short-acting Insulin

Intermediate-acting insulin includes such examples as Neutral Protamine Hagedorn (better known as NPH), Lente, Caninsulin, Humulin N, Novalin N, and, Novolin L (a combination of fast-acting and long-acting insulin). The onset and duration of intermediate-acting insulin is longer and more gradual than short-acting types. Onset varies between 30 minutes and 3 hours. It peaks between 2 and 10 hours. Duration varies from 4 to 24 hours. In many cases, NPH has a shorter duration than Lente insulin, but in some dogs, there seems to be little difference.

Occasionally, Lente or NPH insulin will be prescribed in combination with short-acting types. This is recommended in cases when the intermediate-acting insulin does not have a potent enough action or fast enough onset to regulate a particular pet. Examples might include 50% NPH plus 50% Regular, or 70% NPH plus 30% Regular.

NPH is perhaps the most commonly prescribed insulin for dogs. It usually necessitates two daily injections at 12-hour intervals. Most diabetic dogs and their owners do well on this regime. Be aware, though, that insulin works differently in different dogs. Whereas intermediate-acting insulin lasts 12 hours in *most* dogs, it may last 9, 10, or 13 hours in others.

Long-acting insulin includes Protamine Zinc Insulin (better known as PZI) and Ultralente (or Humulin U). Onset ranges between 1 and 8 hours. Peak action occurs between 4 and 16 hours. Duration can run between 6 and 26 hours.

The benefit of long-acting insulin is the possibility of having to give only a single injection in a 24-hour period. However, possibility is the key word. Ultralente frequently lasts up to 28 hours. If the injection is given at the same time each day, it may result in an overlap of insulin activity. This can be very dangerous for the dog. If an owner is willing to calculate 28-hour intervals, it may be possible to follow a once-a-day injection schedule. Typically, however, long-acting insulin is reserved for use in cats. Dogs are *usually* not well regulated on PZI or Ultralente.

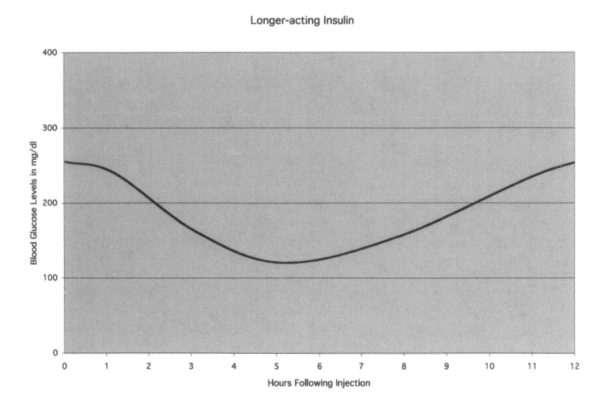

Insulin categorized by source:

A few years ago insulin was available from several different sources. It was possible to find insulin from bovine (beef) sources, porcine (pork) sources, or human sources (synthetic insulin reproduced from human DNA in the laboratory). Diabetic pets typically do very well on animal-based insulin. The molecular structure closely matches their own. Presently these sources are changing.

Animal-based insulin frequently includes the word Iletin in the name. *Iletin I* denotes a combination beef/pork insulin. *Iletin II* is derived entirely from pork sources. Currently, the production of most beef-source insulin, including

Iletin I, is being phased out. The exception to this is PZI. This insulin works so well in cats that it has remained available.

A final example of animal-based insulin is Caninsulin. This insulin is specifically formulated for use in dogs. It is derived from porcine sources and is available in Canada, the United Kingdom, and Australia. It has not been approved for use in the United States.

Unlike most other insulin types, PZI and Caninsulin are formulated in a variety of concentrations (units per cc). Pet owners who administer these types of insulin must be careful to use syringes appropriate to their insulin concentrations.

Human-based insulin is derived from human recombinant DNA, reproduced in a laboratory setting. If the word Humulin appears in the name, the insulin is typically created via bacterial reproduction. If the word Novalin appears in the name, the insulin is produced via yeast reproduction.

Insulin that can be formulated from multiple sources:
Some insulin types can be derived from *either* animal sources or human sources. PZI and NPH are two of these.

Timing meals with injections

To review, unlike diabetes in humans, it is *un*common for dog diabetes to be well-controlled by simply adjusting the diet. Diet does, however, still play an important role in the dog's care.

Chapter 7 described the importance of including high quality, species-appropriate ingredients in the diet. It also discussed the concept of how consistency from meal to meal can be achieved and how this will help regulate a dog's insulin dosage and glucose levels. We will discuss the spacing of meals in this chapter, as it is closely related to insulin activity.

Depending on the type of food, blood sugar begins to rise 1 to 2 hours after a meal is ingested. Diabetic dogs typically do best when they are fed 2, 3, or 4 small meals each day. These dogs maintain more consistent blood sugar levels than those dogs fed only once a day. Severe highs and lows in glucose can be dangerous for your dog. Occasionally, a dog that is a finicky eater may have developed the habit of free-feeding, or nibbling all day long. In most cases it is better to permit this schedule.

The goal in feeding is to ensure that the dog has food in his system when the insulin activity peaks. Dogs receiving two daily insulin injections at 12-hour intervals should also receive two meals at about 12-hour intervals. Dogs receiving only a single insulin injection should receive a main meal prior to that injection, but they, too, will benefit from several more meals spaced throughout the day.

Meals should be offered about 15 minutes prior to the insulin injection. This is a slight departure from the routine followed by human diabetics, but for good reason. Dogs with diabetes often suffer from other digestive complaints. They vomit more readily than do humans. Feeding the meal prior to injection helps ensure that glucose will indeed be available when the insulin activity peaks. If insulin is injected and a dog regurgitates his meal, it could result in dangerously low blood glucose levels. Most dog owners are told to skip an insulin injection if their dog does regurgitate a meal.

Meal Correctly Matched to Insulin Activity

In addition to their main meals, diabetic dogs should also receive several snacks during the day. One snack can be offered midway between breakfast and dinner, and another one, just prior to bedtime. A typical schedule might include breakfast at 7:00 a.m., a snack about noon, dinner at 7:00 p.m., and another small snack before bedtime. If your family is away during the day, consider asking a friend or neighbor to drop by to offer the dog a snack.

These feeding schedules are not set in stone, however. Since each dog responds differently to treatment, adjustments in feeding schedules and insulin injections are common. Your schedule or your dog's metabolism may require you to provide meals and insulin closer together, or farther apart, than the average.

Discuss your needs and questions with your veterinarian. He should be able to tell you (by performing a blood glucose curve test) the length of duration insulin achieves in your particular dog. If you begin home-testing your dog's blood glucose, you will be able to ascertain this information for yourself. The following concepts may be particularly helpful when you want to sleep later on weekend days or when changes in daylight saving's time occur.

Schedule flexibility: insulin duration of 12 hours or less

In cases where insulin *lasts 12 hours or less* in a dog, many owners move a meal one hour or so in either direction without problem. The key is to still provide the injection about 15 minutes after the meal. When this rule of thumb is followed, some veterinarians believe it is acceptable to move the meal up to 2 to 3 hours off schedule, if needed.

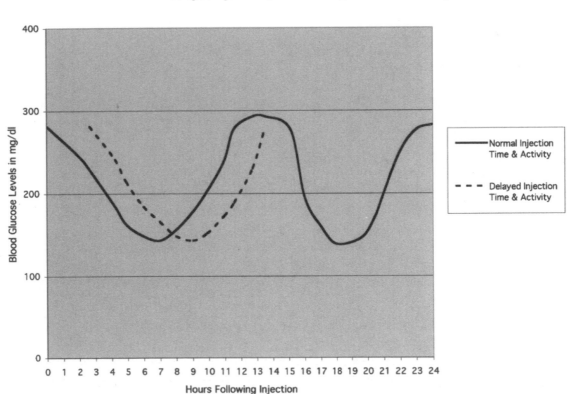

Delayed Injection (Insulin Lasting 12 Hours or Less)

Schedule flexibility: insulin duration greater than 12 hours

In cases where insulin *lasts longer than 12 hours* in a dog, the rule of thumb changes. If insulin is given *too early*, the effects of the current injection will overlap the effects of the previous injection. This can cause a dangerous dip in blood glucose.

To counteract this, many dog owners *slightly reduce the amount* of insulin they are about to inject. Discuss this option with your veterinarian. He may recommend that you reduce it by 10% to 20%, based on how early your schedule requires you to give the injection.

If your schedule requires that you *delay* a greater-than-12-hour injection, you must be aware of these effects, too. If a dog owner promptly returns to the normal schedule after a giving a delayed injection, there is a chance that effects of the delayed injection will overlap the effects of the upcoming one. Again, this can cause a dangerous hypoglycemic episode.

To avoid this dilemma, dog owners often delay the following meals/injections by *a portion* of the original delay time, too. In this way, they avoid a significant overlap of insulin action. Over the course of a few days, these owners have worked their way back up to the original injection and feeding times.

Another option is to *slightly reduce the amount* of insulin that follows the delayed dose, and give it at the normal time. Again, discuss this option with your veterinarian. He may recommend that you reduce it by 10% to 20%, based on the length of the original delay.

Insulin Bottles and Label Information

Insulin is usually dispensed in small, 10 cc glass bottles. The top of the bottle is capped with a rubber stopper and is covered with a metal or plastic outer cap. This maintains the insulin's integrity during distribution and storage at the pharmacy. The outer cap is removed when you are ready to draw up the first injection.

The bottle's label contains some important information. Obviously, the name and strength of the insulin will be printed here, as well as the name of the manufacturer. The label will also include the product outdate, the date until which the insulin will be most effective.

Insulin is available in several different strengths/concentrations. The most common concentration is 100 units of insulin in 1 cc of solution. This is abbreviated U-100. Other concentrations include U-50, which contains 50 units of insulin per cc of solution, and U-40, which contains 40 units of insulin per cc of solution.

If the strength of your dog's insulin has been diluted (with solution being added per your veterinarian's orders) it is important to include this information on the label. This is especially important should your dog (and his insulin) ever be taken to an emergency clinic without you being present.

Syringes and Needles

Unlike other syringes you may have seen, those designed for insulin are especially thin and have a needle permanently attached. As with other syringes, however, they consist of a barrel and a plunger. The barrel is marked off in dosage amounts. The plunger is the portion that expels the liquid.

Both needles and syringes are available in a variety of sizes. Syringes are measured in cubic centimeters (cc's) or milliliters (ml's). These terms are interchangeable. Common syringe sizes include 1 cc, 1/2 cc, 1/3 cc, and 1/4 cc. Small doses of insulin are best prepared in small syringes. The dosage marks are more easily read on smaller syringes. This results in fewer dosage errors.

Needles can vary by length and gauge (diameter.) Common insulin needles include 1/2 inch, 5/8 inch, and 5/16 inch in length and 28, 29, and 30 gauge thickness. A high gauge number refers to a *thinner* needle. Shorter, thinner needles may be more comfortable for small dogs with thin, fragile skin. In more sturdy dogs or those with thickened skin, thin needles may bend and short needles may not insert deep enough into the tissue. Once you find a needle that works for you and your dog, stay with it.

Syringes are also calibrated in terms of insulin concentration. It is best if you administer U-100 insulin with a U-100 syringe, in which one unit of insulin corresponds exactly with each mark on the syringe. Likewise, it is best to administer U-50 insulin with a U-50 syringe and U-40 insulin with a U-40 syringe. Some dog owners have difficulty special ordering U-40 or U-50 syringes, however, and choose to use U-100 syringes instead.

If you do administer insulin *other than* U-100 in a U-100 syringe, you will need to mathematically adjust the volume. This conversion is required because the marks on a U-100 syringe refer to, and "expect" that there will be 100 units of insulin in each cc. If, for example, you use a type of insulin that only contains 50 units in each cc, you would have to fill the U-100 syringe with twice the volume. (Twice the normal mark that corresponds with your dog's dose.)

So, if you are using a **U-50 insulin in a U-100 syringe**, multiply your dog's prescribed dose by 2, and fill the U-100 syringe to that mark. For example, if your dog is prescribed 6 units of U-50 insulin, multiply the 6 by 2. The result is 12. If you fill a U-100 syringe to the 12 mark, your dog will receive his correct dose of 6 units of U-50.

Dose of U-50 _____ x 2 = _____ mark on a U-100 syringe

If you are using **U-40 insulin in a U-100 syringe** multiply your dog's prescribed dose by **2.5** and fill the U-100 syringe to that mark. For example, if your dog is prescribed 6 units of U-40 insulin, multiply the 6 by 2.5. The result is 15. If you fill a U-100 syringe to the 15 mark, your dog will receive his correct dose of 6 units of U-40.

Dose of U-40 _____ x 2.5 = _____ marks on U-100 syringe

If you do administer U-40 or U-50 insulin in a U-100 syringe, do not discuss your dog's dosage in terms of the marks on the syringe. They do not apply to your dog's actual dose. Make sure you understand the difference, in this case, between syringe marks and actual insulin doses.

Reusing Needles and Syringes

Opinion is divided as to whether it is acceptable to reuse insulin needles and syringes. It is common to find arguments and expert recommendations for both cases. As many as 50% of dog owners reuse insulin needles and syringes. This is also a common practice in human healthcare. Repeated use can help reduce the costs of treating this disease.

Dog owners who do reuse syringes only use them a maximum of two times, typically for a morning injection and an evening injection. After passing through skin and fur, the needle is really not *sterile* any longer, but should be considered *clean*. Infection at the injection site does not seem to be a problem in these cases; however, it is always a possibility.

Between injections, the syringe should be stored in a clean Tupperware-type container, in the refrigerator, with the needle pointing upward. This method helps prevent any residual insulin crystals from accumulating in the needle. Do not attempt to clean the needle with alcohol, as it may remove the needle's smooth Teflon coating. This can result in a less comfortable injection.

Other sources, particularly the needle manufacturers, do not recommend needle reuse at all. Microscopic photography demonstrates that needles deteriorate and become dull with each succeeding use. Today's thinner needles bend and torque. If twisted far enough, the tip may break off within the tissue. If yours is a dog that is sensitive to the injection, consider using a needle only once.

Syringe Disposal

In most places, disposal of medical waste (syringes and needles) must follow prescribed guidelines. The specifics differ from state to state and country to country. In many places, it is illegal to simply throw away needles and syringes with your regular garbage. Your veterinarian or sanitation service can provide you with details.

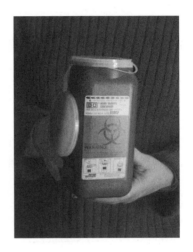

In areas where special medical waste disposal is required, dog owners may use a prefabricated plastic "sharps" container. (Sharps is the medical term for needles and scalpel blades.) These can be obtained through your veterinary clinic, and in many cases, returned there when full. To cut costs, some dog owners economize by using empty, plastic juice or milk jugs, taped closed when full.

Insulin Storage and Handling

Most experts recommend refrigerating insulin at home and even during travel. Some dog owners store their bottles of insulin on their side, on the shelf of the refrigerator door. This method keeps the insulin from separating and requires less mixing prior to injection. Storing insulin in its original box, or in a Tupperware container on the refrigerator's top shelf helps protect it from potential food spills.

Some veterinarians recommend storing insulin in the closed butter compartment of the refrigerator. This keeps the insulin slightly warmer and may result in a more comfortable injection. Many dog owners further warm the insulin by holding the syringe in their fist for a few minutes. Do not use hot water or the microwave to warm insulin. These methods can alter the medication's molecular structure.

Some sources maintain that opened bottles of insulin may be stored out of the refrigerator, but away from bright light. Insulin deteriorates in extreme temperatures and should be discarded if it has been exposed to freezing temperatures or those above 85 degrees F. (30 degrees C.) Other reasons to discard insulin include the presence of white particulate that does not disappear with mixing, insulin that is especially slow to mix, or insulin that sticks to the side of the bottle.

Many sources recommend that insulin be discarded 30 days after opening the bottle. A good deal of controversy exists over this, though. Many dog owners completely finish a bottle of insulin, even if it takes more than a month to do so. They report no noticeable decline in drug action. Recent studies seem to confirm this. All sources *do* recommend discarding insulin once it has reached its printed outdate.

Most diabetic-dog owners keep at least one backup bottle of insulin on hand. Some owners leave a little bit of insulin in the old bottle when they start a new one. This is a safety measure in case they drop and break the new bottle, or they realize there is something wrong with it, once opened. Store unopened bottles in the refrigerator and use the oldest bottle first.

Be sure to keep aware of your dog's insulin supply and plan ahead when ordering. Keep in mind that your veterinarian may be unavailable on holidays and during vacations. In such cases, it may be possible to secure insulin through a veterinary school or emergency clinic.

Preparing Injections

Insulin must be mixed prior to injection by slowly rolling the insulin bottle back and forth, between your palms. Properly mixed insulin will have a cloudy appearance. Improperly mixed insulin will separate and may be ineffective. Insulin should never be shaken or vigorously agitated. This can damage it.

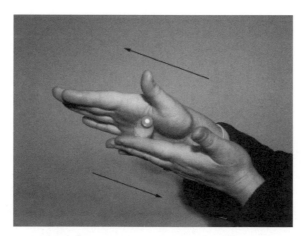

Most dog owners are taught *not* to wipe their dog's skin prior to injection. Considering that the needle must pass through a thick fur coat, insulin injection is really not a sterile procedure. If you do use rubbing alcohol, be certain it has dried prior to injection.

Bottled medications, such as insulin, are prepared under vacuum pressure. As insulin is continually withdrawn from the bottle, the vacuum effect may in-

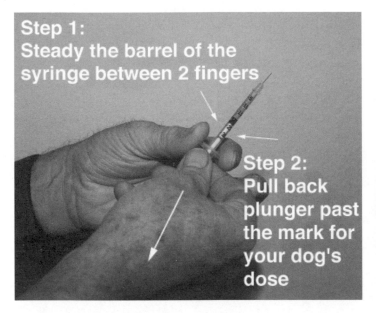

Step 1:
Steady the barrel of the syringe between 2 fingers

Step 2: Pull back plunger past the mark for your dog's dose

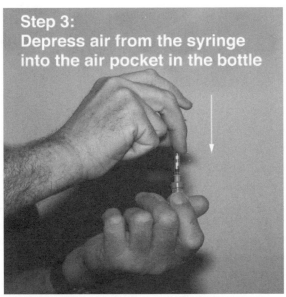

Step 3:
Depress air from the syringe into the air pocket in the bottle

crease. This makes it difficult to withdraw any more insulin. To counteract this effect, inject a small amount of air into the bottle prior to drawing up the insulin. This amount should equal the amount of insulin to be drawn out. If this is done each time, the vacuum pressure will not increase.

To prepare an insulin injection, draw back the plunger of the syringe until you reach the mark that indicates your dog's insulin dose. Insert the needle through the rubber stopper and inject the air into the air-pocket portion of the bottle. Try not to inject air into the insulin, itself. Now you are ready to draw up the insulin.

Invert the bottle so the stopper points toward the floor. Slowly and gently pull back on the plunger. (You will likely have to hold the barrel of the syringe

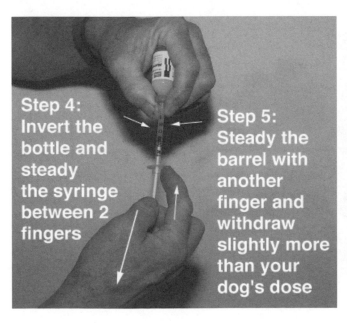

Step 4: Invert the bottle and steady the syringe between 2 fingers

Step 5: Steady the barrel with another finger and withdraw slightly more than your dog's dose

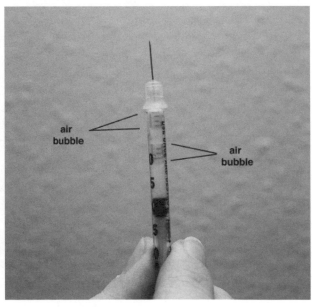

air bubble

air bubble

steady with your other fingers to keep the needle inside the bottle.) Fill the syringe a little past your dog's prescribed dose. It is likely that a few tiny air bubbles will have entered the syringe, and the extra insulin you have drawn up will be used to expel them.

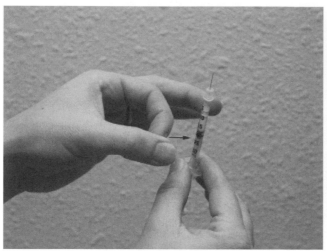 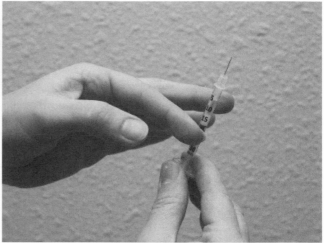

Remove the syringe from the bottle and tap the syringe with a flick from your forefinger. This should cause air bubbles to rise to the top of the syringe. If this is not sufficient, you may choose to expel the entire contents of the syringe back into the bottle and start again. Air bubbles are best removed from the syringe, but avoid agitating the insulin in a prolonged attempt to remove them.

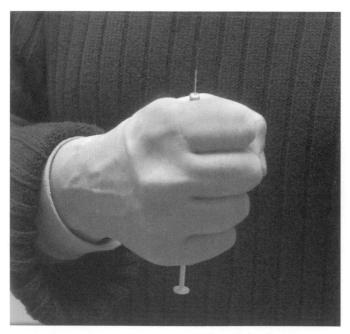

Once the air bubbles have risen to the top of the syringe, depress the plunger until you reach the mark on the syringe that represents your dog's prescribed dose. If you have difficulty seeing the marks on the syringe, purchase a tabletop magnifying glass. This style allows you to keep both hands free. They are available at pharmacies. Be sure good lighting is available, as well.

Once you are sure you have drawn up the correct dose, warm the insulin by holding the syringe in your fist for a moment. Be very careful to avoid touching and contaminating the sterile needle. Some dog owners draw up the injection an hour or two prior to injection time, set it in a safe place, out of direct sunlight, and allow the syringe to come to room temperature by itself.

Some dogs' insulin doses differ between their morning and evening injections. If your dog is supposed to receive one particular dose in the morning and *a different dose* in the evening, be conscious of drawing-up the correct amount at the correct time.

If your dog's prescription requires you to **draw up two different types of insulin** in the same syringe, the procedure is slightly different. Beginning with the short-acting insulin (R), inject the quantity of air into that bottle that represents your dog's dose of *that* insulin. Don't withdraw any insulin yet. Withdraw the needle.

Next, switch to the bottle of longer-acting insulin. Inject the quantity of air into the bottle that represents your dog's dose of *that* insulin. This time, fill the syringe with insulin slightly past your dog's dosage mark. Tap the syringe to loosen any air bubbles. Expel the bubbles and any excess insulin until you reach the dog's correct dosage of the longer-acting insulin.

Finally, switch back to the bottle of short-acting insulin (R). Insert the needle, and being careful not to push any of the longer-acting insulin into the bottle, withdraw the appropriate amount of the short-acting insulin (R). Do not try to expel any more air bubbles at this point.

If it will be a few moments before you will actually give the injection (you must call the dog in the house, or prepare his meal), you may very carefully recap the needle, or rest it in such a way that the needle will remain sterile. Nothing must touch it, and it must not roll anywhere and touch something else. If it does, discard that syringe and insulin and prepare a fresh one.

Pre-filling Syringes and Enlisting the Help of Others

It is possible to prepare insulin injections well in advance (several weeks) of when they will be needed. This is valuable if you are taking the dog on a trip, or leaving him in the care of someone trained in injection technique. A few hints can help the process go smoothly.

If your dog receives insulin that differs in dosage between his morning and evening injection, label these carefully. Place a piece of tape around the barrel, leaving a flag on which to write. Avoid covering the dosage markings that are applicable to your dog's dose. Perhaps the most foolproof way to label syringes is by simply printing "morning, ___ cc's" and "evening, ___ cc's" on the tape.

Pre-drawn syringes should be stored in a clean Tupperware-type container in the refrigerator. They should be stored with the needle end facing up, to minimize the chance of insulin crystals accumulating in the needle.

The insulin in pre-drawn syringes must be mixed again, just prior to injection. The syringe should be held with the needle pointing upward between the palms and gently rolled back and forth.

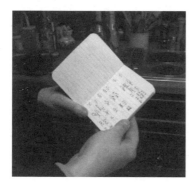

Written notes can also help minimize communication errors. Have a small notebook or calendar available for the dog's caretaker or yourself if you are travelling with your dog. Jotting down the time and insulin dose will help avoid double doses and clear up questions that might arise, especially if the dog has an unusual reaction.

Giving Insulin Injections

The thought of giving a pet a hypodermic injection can be daunting. Most often there is a fear of causing the pet pain. A brief education and some manual practice can greatly reduce this concern. Once you have read through the procedure a few times, and practiced with your dog, it will be much less intimidating. Within a short time, injections will become a normal part of the day for both you and your dog.

Locating and Rotating Injection Sites

Historically, dogs have been given most vaccines at the scruff of their neck. The underlying tissue may be thickened and somewhat scarred in this area. Consequently, this is *not* a good location for insulin injections. Insulin may be absorbed unreliably from scarred areas.

Instead, owners are commonly taught to use the sides of the dog's neck, the shoulder blade area and the hips (when the dog is seated). Actually, any spot where you can lift up the skin will probably suffice. Individual dogs differ in their anatomy and sensitivity. Avoid areas in which your dog seems ticklish.

Once you have decided on a general area that works well for both you and your dog, rotate injection sites by about an inch for each injection. You may also rotate from one side of the dog's body, to the other side.

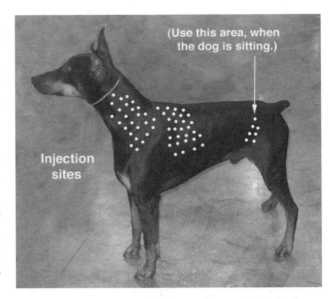

(Use this area, when the dog is sitting.)

Injection sites

If you notice the general area becomes thickened or lumpy, change to a different area of the dog's body. Be aware, however, that moving to a completely new area may result in different insulin absorption rates. Watch your dog's behavior if you change injection sites by more than a couple of inches.

Procedure Description

Insulin is normally injected in the subcutaneous layer, the fatty area between the skin and underlying muscle. You may hear veterinary staff refer to this as "sub-Q" or see it abbreviated as SQ. The sub-Q area is located by pulling up the dog's fur in the shape of a tent. By doing this, the skin is broadly separated from the underlying muscle. This creates easy access to the subcutaneous area.

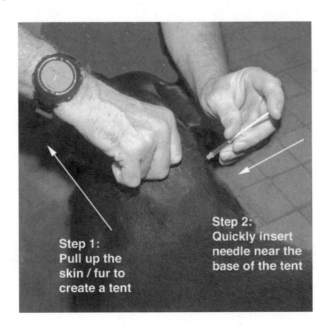

Step 1: Pull up the skin / fur to create a tent

Step 2: Quickly insert needle near the base of the tent

Most owners do not use alcohol wipes on the dog's skin. Considering that the needle must pass through a thick fur coat, it is questionable as to whether injecting a dog is a sterile procedure. If, however, a dog is thoroughly muddy from a day in the field, it may be advisable to locate a different injection site and schedule a bath.

There are several different methods for handling the syringe. Practice them all and decide which is most comfortable for you. In the first method, the syringe is held like a dart, between the thumb, index finger, and third finger, palm facing the dog. Once the needle is inserted, the owner quickly repositions his hand by flipping his palm upward and re-grasping the barrel between his index finger and third finger (like a cigarette). The thumb is placed on the plunger and injects the insulin. Because the thumb is a strong finger, this method offers good control in delivering the insulin smoothly and quickly. Do not release your hold on the tent, however, as you attempt to reposition your syringe hand. If you find it necessary to drop the tent, try a different method.

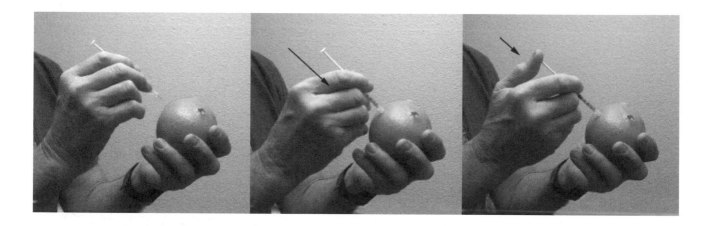

In the second method, the syringe is held between the thumb and third finger, with the index finger held above the plunger, palm facing the dog. Once the syringe is inserted, the index finger may contact the plunger and express the insulin. If the index finger rests on the plunger *during* insertion, insulin may be expelled too early.

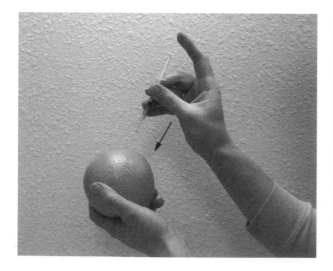
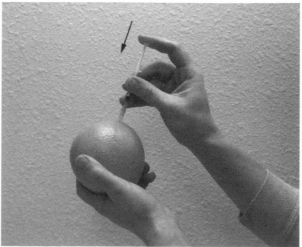

The third method of injection involves holding the syringe like a cigarette, between the index finger and the third finger, knuckles facing the dog. The injection is made in a backhanded motion. Once inserted, the thumb is placed on the plunger and the insulin is injected. These last two methods are good in cases where dogs fidget, since they do not require you to reposition your hand.

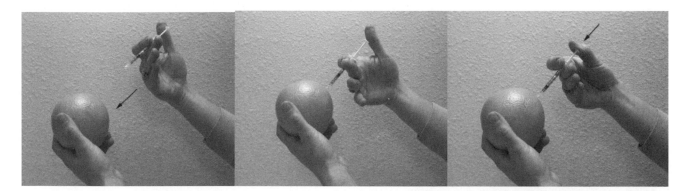

Aim for the broad area of the tent, close to the dog's body. If you aim for the narrower portions at the top of the tent, the needle may exit through the skin on the other side and the insulin will be injected out *onto* the fur, not *into* the subcutaneous space. This is one of the most common ways to have an injection go wrong.

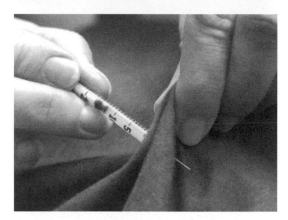

With the fur pulled up in your nondominant hand and the syringe in your dominant hand, completely insert the needle into the tented area. Use a firm, smooth motion, with conviction, rather like throwing a dart. A quick and smooth insertion is more comfortable for the patient than a slow and timid insertion.

Depending on how you have decided to hold the syringe, move your fingers, if necessary, and smoothly depress the plunger. Remove the needle quickly. Do not rub or massage the injection site as this may alter the action of the insulin. Do, by all means, give the dog a pat or hug in a different area of his body.

Practicing Injections – the Dog Owner's Part

It is helpful to practice injection technique before actually performing it on the dog. In fact, it is best practiced without the dog even present. We will discuss the dog's part in the upcoming section.

You may practice on a stuffed animal, a pillow, or a piece of fruit or chicken. Take an empty syringe and fill it either with insulin or just with air. Review the various options for holding the syringe. Start with the option that seems most comfortable to you. With your nondominant hand, pretend to pull up the skin in a tent.

Insert the needle quickly and with confidence. Remember that you should aim for the lower part of the tent. Smoothly and gradually depress the plunger. Quickly remove the needle and give the pillow, fruit, or stuffed toy a hug and a pretend food treat. Remember that you should not rub the actual injection site.

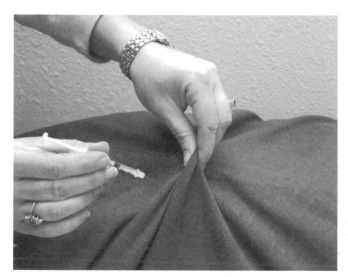 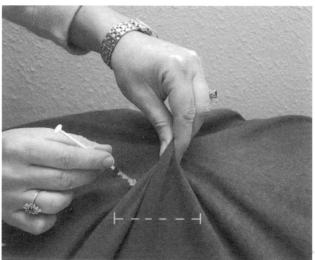

As you become more comfortable with your technique, also practice talking to your pet. Many pet owners keep up a calm running banter during the injection procedure. This is enormously reassuring to dogs. What you actually say is far less important than the tone you use. Also remember to dispose of any syringes you use for practice.

Training for Injections – the Dog's Part

You might also find it helpful to give your dog a few *pretend* injections. Since you know it will be just practice, you will be less likely to experience feelings of anxiety. Consequently, your dog will be less likely to read these emotions in you. Instead, you can help him view the whole experience as a rewarding interaction.

Before you begin, place several (5 to 10) food treats on a plate or tray. These can be very small morsels of whatever type of food agrees with your dog. Small bits of cooked, low-fat meat, such as chicken or turkey, are good choices. Even the most finicky eaters will usually not turn down small flakes of tuna fish. You may also use a favorite toy or game as a reward.

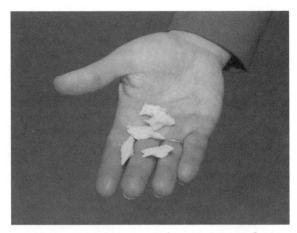

In addition to the food treats or toy, set out the insulin bottle and a syringe. It can be helpful to let the dog see these items during a practice session. Eliminate loud television or radio noises, and make sure your practice area is well lit. Put other pets outdoors or in another room for a few moments so you can practice without interference. Try to limit family member interruptions as well. Remember: Everything about this practice session should be fun for the dog.

Begin by massaging or grooming your pet with a brush. This type of activity is believed to release endorphins (chemicals in the brain) that act as a natural painkiller. Work your way up to the dog's shoulder blade area (or other area you plan to use).

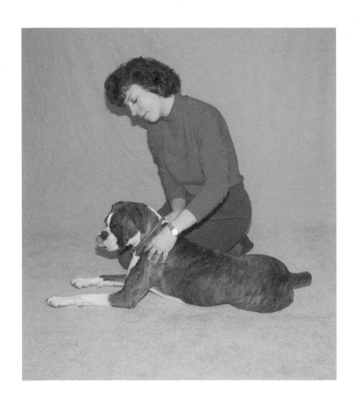

Lift up his skin on his shoulder to form a tent. Be careful not to squeeze too hard as you lift the tent. Release the skin, give him a food treat, and tell him how good he is.

Next, lift up the skin again and push your dominant index finger against the tent in the area you would inject. Release the skin and offer him another treat. If your dog seems apprehensive about your activities, offer him verbal reassurance and continue this exercise until he relaxes.

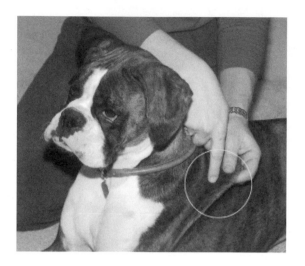 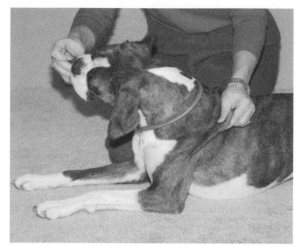

Eventually, he will begin to view your activities as pleasant and rewarding. During actual injections, many owners have found it helpful to place the food treat where dog can see or smell it. Their dogs are usually very well-behaved in anticipation of their reward.

If yours is a high energy, active dog, you may need to distract him during this practice session. If he has been obedience trained, put him on either a sit-stay or a down-stay (discussed in the upcoming section). If he cannot perform this exercise, you may distract him with a meal. This is helpful when a dog tries to turn around to see what you are doing, or attempts to avoid your touch.

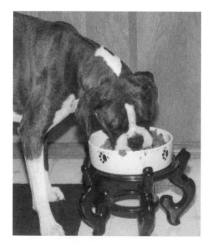

Place his food bowl down. It may be helpful to feed your dog from a raised food bowl, so that the skin around the dog's shoulder blades is relaxed and not pulled taught. As he begins to eat, practice making the tent. Since he is already eating, you may substitute verbal praise as his reward. Praise him in calm, drawn-out words and phrases. "Goo-o-o-d dog." Keep the tone of your voice low.

Once your dog is familiar and relaxed with the injection practice, allow him to smell (not lick) the insulin bottle and capped syringe. These items will have distinct smells to the dog and allowing him to smell them now will remove one more element of unfamiliarity when it comes time for the actual injection. Many dogs will be unimpressed with these items.

Teaching the Dog to Stay

You might find it helpful to have your dog sit or lie still for his insulin injection. If he has not been trained in these exercises or he needs a refresher course, this can be readily accomplished by using a canine instinct called the oppositional reflex. This describes the tendency to pull back or pull away from tension. It is a very effective method of teaching a dog to stay in place.

Teach and practice the sit or down-stay separate from injection time. A good time to practice this is later in the evening when energetic dogs typically calm down. When the dog can hold a sit-stay or down-stay for just a few moments, you can incorporate it into your injection technique.

Choose a quiet setting in which to work. Prepare a small supply of food treats and place them close at hand: your pocket, the edge of a table or countertop, or even tucked inside your cheek. Place a leash and collar on your dog. Do not use choke chain or prong collars for teaching the stay; instead, use a wide, flat, buckle-type collar.

The Sit-Stay: With one hand, place gentle pressure on the dog's rump and/or raise the treat back and over his head. These motions should encourage the dog into a sitting position. Once in this position, allow him to eat the food treat. With one hand on his rump and the other hand on the leash, about six inches from the collar, gradually pull forward on the leash *and* gently press down against his rump.

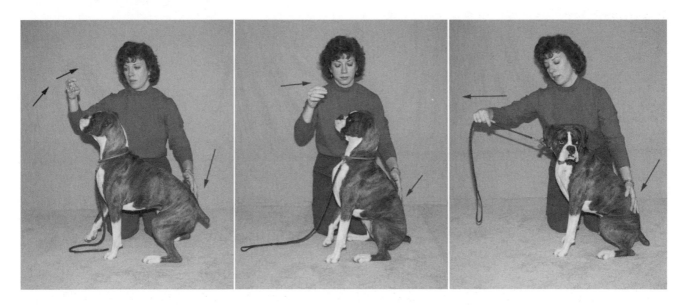

The pressure on the collar should produce the oppositional reflex. As you pull the leash forward, the dog *should* pull backward, cementing himself in the sit position. Tell him, "Sta-a-ay."

Occasionally, a submissive dog will attempt to get up and following the leash pressure. If this begins to happen, quickly increase pressure on the dog's rump to keep him from rising. When he resumes the sit position, tell him, "Sta-a-ay." Give him a food treat. Bring the food treat quickly to his mouth so that he does not try to reach for it and stand up.

With time, he will begin to oppose the pressure on the collar. You can increase the duration, a few moments at a time, before you offer him the treat.

The Down-Stay: The method of teaching the down-stay is very similar. The main difference is that you will initially position the dog by leading his nose down to the floor with the food treat in your hand. Simultaneously put gentle but steady pressure along his spine.

Once the dog is in the down position, the procedure is essentially the same. Put forward pressure on the leash while maintaining the down position with your other hand on the dog's back or shoulders.

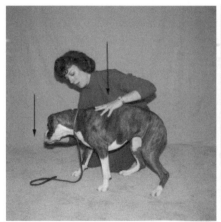 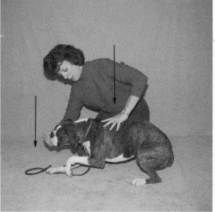 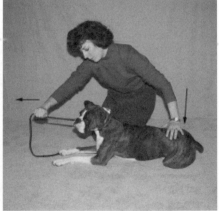

Injections Gone Wrong / Complications

Once you have practiced with your dog, you should be more prepared to actually give him his insulin injections. Naturally, it will be a different experience than the practice situations and you may have some injections that don't go as planned.

If the syringe begins to fill with blood after insertion, it means the needle has entered a blood vessel. It is best not to inject insulin directly into the bloodstream, as it would greatly accelerate the expected action. Withdraw the needle and reinsert it an inch or two away from the first site. Be certain you are lifting up the skin to create the tent effect.

If, after depressing the plunger, you see or feel a wet spot in the dog's fur or your hand, it indicates that the dog did not receive some or all of his insulin. The safest course of action is to do nothing. This may result in increased blood glucose levels, but the rise will likely be for only a day or so.

The option of "doing nothing" is much safer than trying to estimate how much insulin was injected and then re-injecting more. If too much insulin is given, your dog could experience a dangerous episode of hypoglycemia (low blood sugar.) A faulty injection is nothing to be upset about. Even the most experienced dog owners occasionally have an injection that goes wrong.

If you do miss an injection, because of shipment delays, technique, or other reason, it is not an emergency. Missing an occasional single dose will not likely cause your dog much harm. During this time, though, you might notice the signs of polyuria and polydipsia return. Prepare for this by having ample drinking water available, offering extra trips outside, and placing washable padding in or around your dog's bed.

Occasionally, a dog will yelp or wince upon injection. Diabetic-dog owners believe this is a very individual matter, most likely related to a particular dog's anatomy and nerve pathways. Human diabetics report that the discomfort is minor and passes quickly. In such cases, you may either continue with the injection, or reposition the needle and finish the injection in another spot. If your dog seems extremely pained by insulin injections, you can rub a bit of infant-teething anesthetic on the skin, prior to injection time.

Once in a while an injection will result in a lump at the injection site. While it may feel and look alarming, such a lump does not usually present a problem and will resolve itself in several days. Human diabetics experience these lumps, as well.

Some owners give the injection while the dog is eating. This can act as both a distraction *and* a reward to the dog. This method does carry with it the risk of having the dog regurgitate after the insulin has been given, however, so it is best used with reliable eaters. This method is not advised for use with finicky eaters.

Until injections become part of your normal routine, it may be helpful to have a system to keep track of when injections are given. This might include a notebook or marks on a calendar. Some owners who reuse syringes use the syringe itself as a visual cue as to whether an injection has been given. They know that if the empty syringe is in the refrigerator, the morning shot was given. If the syringe is still in the refrigerator by early evening, they know they have not yet given the evening injection.

If more than one individual in the house gives injections, written notes on a calendar or journal can help avoid double dosing the dog. Some families recommend the practice of putting one individual in charge of diabetes care. In other words, one person is responsible for giving meals and injections unless other family members are specifically requested to do so.

In the absence of such a routine, errors like insulin overdose can occur. Overdose can also be caused by distractions while drawing up the injection, or by a helper or pet-sitter who does not completely understand the procedure. If the overdose is minor, additional food and a phone call to the veterinarian are in order. If the overdose is significant, immediately take the dog, along with Karo syrup and a helper/family member, to the nearest veterinary clinic. This is a serious situation. Hypoglycemic effects can last for several days, and it is best if the dog is hospitalized overnight.

Hypoglycemic Incidents

The condition of hypoglycemia is a serious side effect of giving insulin. (To help remember the definition of hypoglycemia, remember that hypo rhymes with "low.") It is usually defined as a blood glucose level less than 60 mg/dl or 3.29 mmol/L. (Normal glucose levels range between 65 mg/dl and 120 mg/dl.)

Signs of hypoglycemia can, unfortunately, seem very much like those of *hyper*glycemia. They may include behavior changes such as restlessness *or* lethargy, disorientation, being glassy-eyed or staring off into space, muscle weakness, wobbliness, or lack of coordination, changes in appetite, shivering, perspiring paws, seizures, and coma. Dogs may vary in their symptoms. This depends on how rapidly and how far glucose levels drop. Also, the same dog can exhibit different symptoms from one hypoglycemic episode to another.

Interestingly, however, some dogs can experience low blood glucose levels *without* manifesting any unusual signs. This is known as asymptomatic hypoglycemia. Some dogs can have glucose levels as low as 20 mg/dl or 30 mg/dl without any of the usual hypoglycemic signs. With time, you will learn to read your dog's behaviors and anticipate his needs.

Since episodes of hypoglycemia — also called hypo events — can come unexpectedly, it is important for dog owners to be prepared in advance. You can accomplish this by having emergency sources of glucose available in your house, car, and when you go for walks.

There are commercial glucose tablets and glucagon injections available for human diabetics, but a more effective and economical option for pet owners is to use some form of liquid sugar. Dog owners have found Karo syrup (a high fructose corn syrup found with baking supplies in United States markets), maple syrup, and pancake syrup very effective in raising the blood glucose level (bgs). Many of these syrups are available in small packets that can be kept in the car, barn/workshop, or attached to the dog's leash. These packets can be found at many fast food restaurants. Some dog owners use small tubes of cake frosting with equal success.

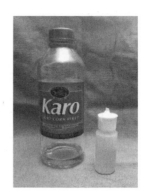

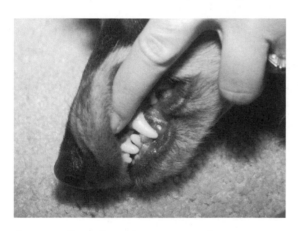

When a dog does experience a hypo event, owners should immediately lift the dog's lips and rub the syrup inside his cheeks and along the gums. Glucose is quickly absorbed from mucous membranes in the mouth. If your dog is experiencing stupor, seizure, or lack of coordination, do not try to get the dog to swallow the syrup, as it may cause him to choke. If your dog is staggering, help him lie down.

Once the dog is more alert, you may wish to let him lick up a bit more of the syrup. Many dog owners use the following rule of thumb: 1 to 2 tablespoons per 10 pounds of body weight. Shortly afterward, offer the dog a snack. The effects of the sugar last only a short time and dogs in this situation benefit from a longer-term rise in blood glucose, as well.

It is important to discuss this plan with your veterinarian before it should occur. Share this plan with your family members or pet-sitter. You may even find it helpful to print and post these instructions in a readily accessible place, such as a bulletin board or on the refrigerator. Include the phone numbers of your regular veterinary clinic and after-hours emergency clinic. Make sure the syrup is always located in a specific place so that any family member can find it at any time. It is easy for dog owners to become distraught during such an event and a prepared plan can be helpful.

Place a call to your veterinarian or veterinary emergency clinic and explain the hypoglycemic event. The staff will want to know how the dog is reacting. If your dog has experienced a seizure or period of unconsciousness, you will be instructed to bring him to the clinic.

Your veterinarian may likely instruct you to reduce one or more of the dog's upcoming insulin doses (usually by 10% to 20%). A full dose might send the dog back into hypoglycemia. Serious cases of hypoglycemia may require that the following dose of glucose be skipped entirely.

Owners who test their dog's blood glucose at home can report this information to their veterinarian and use it to adjust the following insulin doses appropriately. In fact, the experience of a having a hypoglycemic event is what motivates many dog owners to begin home blood testing.

Continue to monitor your dog for signs of hypoglycemia. The insulin may be very active and may continue to lower blood glucose levels even after you have provided emergency treatment. If you know the general activity of your dog's insulin, you can better treat hypo events. (For example, if you know that the insulin will continue to lower blood glucose for another few hours, you will realize how important it is to offer him an additional snack after the syrup. Support his blood sugar until the peak insulin activity has passed.) It can take some dogs several hours or even a day to return to their normal behaviors.

Other circumstances that may warrant hypo treatment (syrup on the gums) can include the following: when a dog vomits after you have given him his insulin injection, or if you think you have injected into the bloodstream. In the case of the latter, review your technique to avoid this in the future. Watch your dog's behavior when you start a new bottle of insulin. Some dogs tend to experience low glucose levels in this situation.

One dog owner, living on a large farm, outfitted her dog with a glow-in-the-dark collar and bell. Since her dog is a working farm dog, these measures will help her locate the dog should he ever become disoriented or difficult to find. Other owners have purchased or have had special collar tags made. They include the message that the dog is a diabetic and receives insulin, along with the name and phone number of the veterinary clinic.

Regulating Glucose Levels

Diabetic-dog owners quickly become familiar with the goal of getting their pet regulated. This term means that blood glucose levels and clinical signs are effectively controlled for the greater part of the day. When a dog becomes regulated, symptoms such as polydipsia and polyuria typically decline, appetite decreases, and body weight usually stabilizes.

Theoretically, dogs can be considered regulated when their blood glucose levels run between 65 mg/dl and 120 mg/dl; however, achieving such tight control can be difficult with dogs. It is partly a safety issue. Dogs cannot tell us when they feel hypoglycemic and many owners are not at home around the clock to deal with such a potential event. In addition, it can be difficult to control a dog's behavior. He may be active one day or sleep soundly, another.

Therefore, some veterinarians and dog owners refer to a more realistic rule of thumb. They try to maintain diabetic dogs *without* cataracts between 100 mg/dl (5.49 mmol/L) and 200 mg/dl (10.99 mmol/L). Dogs with cataracts are maintained between 100 mg/dl and 250 mg/dl. (Since lower bgs may help forestall cataract development, tight control may be eased once cataracts have developed.)

*Un*regulated dogs continue to experience blood glucose levels that are too high *or* too low. High glucose levels, or hyperglycemia, can cause severe damage over time. Signs can include sluggish behavior, slow movements, sleepiness *or* restlessness, depression, isolation, polydipsia, polyuria, appetite changes, and the impression that the dog is simply "not feeling well."

There are several approaches to regulating diabetic dogs. In the most conservative approach, the dog's blood glucose is periodically measured at the veterinary hospital and the owners merely keeps track of **clinical signs**. In other cases, owners are encouraged to perform **urine glucose testing**, in addition to monitoring signs. In the most aggressive approach owners **monitor blood glucose levels** at home.

Achieving diabetes regulation is not the same as learning to ride a bike. Once it happens, it doesn't always remain constant. As you will learn, many factors can influence glucose control. Getting and staying regulated is a fluid process that can take many months. And, even once your dog is regulated, a particular type of insulin may demonstrate a different activity than it originally did. A typical dose of insulin is about 0.5 units per kilogram of bodyweight, per *injection* (not, that is, per *day*), but this rate may be adjusted many times as the veterinarian attempts to regulate your dog.

Blood Glucose Testing at the Veterinary Clinic

Shortly after your veterinarian has started your dog on insulin injections, he will likely recommend a blood glucose curve test be performed at the clinic. In fact, if your dog was hospitalized at the time of diagnosis, he may have had a curve performed before he was discharged. This test is performed over an extended time frame, usually 12 or 24 hours, the latter providing a more complete picture of insulin activity.

Your dog will remain at the veterinary clinic during this time. If he does not eat well at the clinic, you may be instructed to feed him at home. An intravenous catheter will be placed in a blood vessel and small blood samples will be withdrawn at one-hour or two-hour intervals to measure glucose levels. When these results are plotted on a graph, a curve develops. The curve demonstrates how well the insulin controls blood glucose and if any adjustments should be made.

This test can be psychologically stressful for both owner and dog, however. Such stress can be reflected in the test results, skewing them somewhat. Blood glucose curves are performed periodically, such as when a particular dose and type of insulin no longer keeps a dog regulated, or when a change in dosage has been made. If no problems seem apparent, your doctor may recommend the test be routinely repeated every 3 to 6 months.

Subjectively Monitoring Clinical Signs

One way of regulating diabetic dogs is to adjust insulin dosages based on the presence or absence of clinical signs, such as polydipsia and polyuria. Your veterinarian may instruct you to monitor and record water consumption and urine volume. This can be done both by counting the number of trips a dog makes to the yard, and the length of time he relieves himself (counting out the duration of a dog's stream).

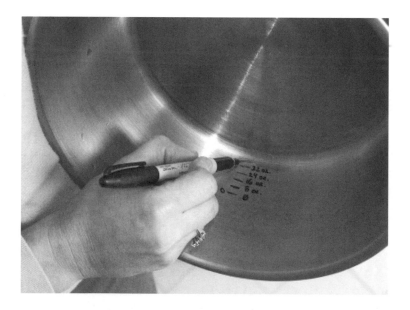

To monitor water intake, mark the inside of the dog's water bowl with a waterproof marking pen, denoting cups, 1/2 cups, 1/4 cups, or even ounces, for small dogs. Keep written records in a small journal or on the calendar. This method may be more reliable than trying to monitor urine output, since a dog with free access to the yard may urinate when you are not watching.

Average daily water consumption is approximately 1 cup of water for every 10 pounds of body weight (or 250 ml for every 4.5 kg of body weight). Dogs eating homemade diets typically drink less. If you have more than one dog, they may need to be separated during the time you are trying to monitor water intake, each with his own water source.

Insulin adjustments are typically made slowly and conservatively. When the signs become controlled, your veterinarian will have you remain with that insulin dosage. If symptoms should return, your veterinarian will likely have you increase your dog's dosage again.

On one hand, this may seem to be an easy, low-maintenance approach to diabetic care, but there are several other aspects to consider. A conservative approach can result in an extended period of *un*regulated diabetes. During this time owners must continually deal with urinary accidents in the house, extra laundry, etc. Long periods of high blood glucose levels also contribute to cataract formation, and internal organ and nerve damage. Also, pets exhibit widely varying clinical signs. Diabetes is known as a silent disease and much can be occurring on the inside of a body that is not visible on the outside.

To know if a dog is truly regulated, *some* form of home glucose testing is recommended. Glucose levels can be tested in several ways. This includes urine testing and blood testing.

Urine Glucose Testing

Since glucose spills into the urine between 180 mg/dl and 220 mg/dl, periodic urine testing can provide information as to how well a dog is regulated. If glucose is present in urine, a dog is *not* well regulated. Such a case would likely require an increased insulin dose or switching to an insulin with a longer duration or more potent action. These are options to discuss with your veterinarian.

Urine glucose testing is performed by dipping a paper test strip into a urine sample. These strips will change color according to the amount of glucose in the urine. Glucose levels are usually read at 30 seconds by comparing the color of the strip to the color range chart printed on the test strip container. Be sure to read the instructions that come with your test strips.

These strips go by several brand names; the most common are Diastix or Clinistix (which test for the presence of glucose only) and Keto-Diastix (which tests for the presence of both glucose and ketones). These strips use very different color scales and measurement scales. Be sure that you and your veterinarian are discussing the same type of test strip and its results.

Many veterinarians recommend collecting the urine sample first thing each morning. Until this becomes a routine habit, plan on leaving yourself some extra time in the morning before leaving for work. In addition, you may be encouraged to test urine glucose levels several other times during the day. Dog owners joke about what their neighbors must think as they run behind their dog each morning. With time, it will just become part of your normal day.

There are several ways to collect a urine sample. The urine sample does not need to be sterile for glucose testing, only "clean." You can use a clean ceramic mug, margarine container, or plastic zip-style bag. Follow the dog into the yard. Walk along with him, but pretend you are not very interested in his activities. Most dogs are accustomed to relieving themselves, *by* themselves, and may be intimidated if their owner follows them around. After the dog squats or lifts his leg, quietly slip the cup or container under the urine stream, once he has started. If he seems especially alarmed by what you are doing, offer him a food treat afterward.

If your aim is poor, and the idea of urine on your hand bothers you, purchase a pair or box of latex gloves. One dog owner used the large half of a pooper-scooper to catch the urine. Another used a soup ladle. This alleviates the need to bend down. With time, the dog will not even notice what you are doing.

Test the urine immediately. Only fresh urine samples should be used for glucose testing. Glucose breaks down quickly and an old urine sample may present a falsely negative glucose test result.

Your veterinarian will likely have instructed you to call him when you have particular results or he may have provided you with instructions on how to make *minor* adjustments to insulin doses based on your test readings. Following are the glucose reading recommendations followed by *one* dog owner using Diastix test strips. Discuss the following sample schedule with your own veterinarian. He may give you instructions to suit your particular pet or he may not wish you to adjust insulin at all without the benefit of a glucose curve.

If the morning dipstick is:	Adjust the insulin by:
Negative	Reduce by 1 unit
1/10	Same dose, no change
1/4	Same dose, no change
1/2	Increase by 1 unit
1	Increase by 1 unit
2	Increase by 1 unit

There *are* several drawbacks to urine testing. First, blood glucose levels must be elevated for an extended period before it spills into the urine. Second, urine testing is not a very accurate form of monitoring glucose levels. It provides a delayed picture of what is occurring within your dog's body. The urine you measure has been stored in the dog's bladder for several hours, even overnight. The measurements reflect glucose levels that have been averaged out over all that time. The longer the urine is stored, the more inaccurate the glucose reading can be. Urine measurements do not indicate how the dog is doing at the moment.

For example, a urine sample taken at midday may indicate that glucose levels are acceptable. That measurement really reflects the glucose metabolism during the course of the morning. In reality, the insulin effect may be wearing off by midday, and your dog may be spending much of his time with very high glucose levels.

In another example, if your dog's evening insulin injection does not have an adequate duration, he may spend much of his evening with high blood glucose levels. The morning urine reading may be quite high, but the morning insulin injection will reduce it. If you were to increase insulin, based on the urine reading, you could bring your dog's glucose level to dangerously low levels. Remember that morning readings really reflect information from hours ago.

The delay in information can be enormously frustrating for dog owners who are having difficulty getting their pets regulated. Traipsing out in the rain and snow to collect a urine sample may quickly lose its charm. Daily events continually affect glucose levels: exercise, an unexpected binge on forbidden food, weight loss or weight gain, psychological stress, concurrent diseases or infections. Finally, urine testing does not indicate whether a dog has had a hypoglycemic episode. These issues combined cause many diabetic-dog owners to consider the benefits of home blood glucose testing. Human diabetics, even children, are taught to monitor their blood glucose levels at home. Many dog owners are following their lead.

Home Blood Glucose Testing

Dog owners monitor their dog's glucose levels to have better control over their dog's disease, cut costs, and avoid hypoglycemic events. In addition, some pets are extremely stressed by a stay at the veterinary clinic. It raises their glucose levels so high that the test results are almost meaningless. Home testing can eliminate this.

Many veterinarians do not support home blood testing. Some are not aware that it is a possibility. Others are apprehensive that dog owners will make irresponsible changes to insulin regimes. If you wish to begin home blood testing, it may be helpful to find a veterinarian who supports you in this pursuit. Many a veterinarian has had a change of heart once a client has successfully and intelligently monitored his dog at home.

Performing home glucose testing can be intimidating to dog owners, just as insulin injections were at first. Read through the procedure several times. Then practice handling the equipment and practice the procedure on a stuffed animal or piece of fruit. If you test it on yourself, remember that human fingers are more sensitive than the prick sites used on dogs. Use the same positive reinforcement training techniques that you have previously used with your dog. Practice the sit or down-stay. Practice a pretend blood stick with pressure from your finger. Reward your dog with food, hugs, or praise. And finally, allow him to smell the equipment.

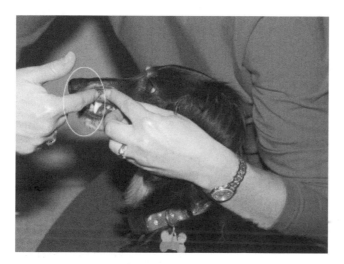
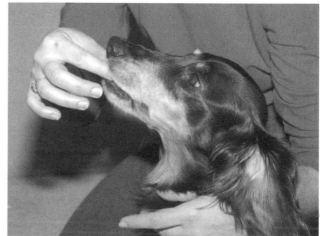

Blood Glucose Testing Equipment

In home glucose testing, a tiny prick is made in the skin with a tool called a **lancet**. The resulting droplet of blood is placed on a paper strip and inserted into a small, handheld machine. In the United States, anyone may purchase blood glucose testing equipment without a prescription. Meters, lancets, and testing strips are available at pharmacies (including budget and warehouse style stores) and over the Internet. If you are uncertain about doing home testing, and worry that your pet may not tolerate it, you can purchase a box of lancets alone, without the meter. Read and practice the procedure for using the lancets, and if all goes well, purchase the meter afterward.

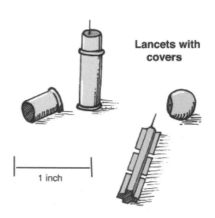

Lancets with covers

1 inch

Lancets are available in a variety of shapes and sizes. Some are quite small and fine, and are good for sensitive individuals. These are shaped like tiny, smooth cones. Others are available with angled edges that may work better on thick-skinned individuals, and those that don't easily bleed. If you don't like the type that comes with meter, you may purchase a different type of lancet separately.

If you experience difficulty obtaining a blood droplet after pricking your dog, be certain you are inserting the lancet forcefully, to its full length. One owner even gives the lancet a half turn to increase blood flow.

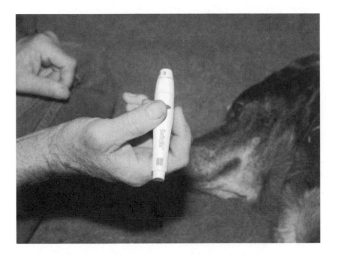

Lancets can be used alone or in conjunction with a firing device or lancet pen. These are button-activated, pen-shaped devices that push the lancet in with a spring action. Some dog owners feel they have better control when using the lancets alone. Others are squeamish about performing the prick and find a firing device helpful. Some sensitive dogs may be frightened by the noise of the firing device.

If using a lancet pen for the first time, start at middle setting and move upwards. Thick-skinned dogs may require the highest settings (deepest prick). Massage the area you are about to prick before placing the pen down. Gently press pen against the tissue before firing it.

Meters (glucometers) are available in numerous styles, but pet owners have a few favorites. These machines do not require that you take the drop of blood to the machine; instead, the machine can be brought to the drop of blood. In these machines, capillary action actually draws-up the blood. This is much easier than having to squeeze a drop of blood onto a test strip.

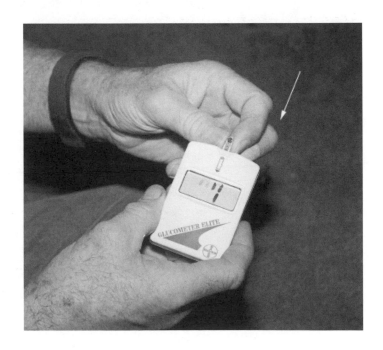

The glucometers most favored by dog owners include:

➤ **Bayer Glucometer Elite** and **Elite XL** – these meters require a smaller blood sample than do most other meters. Owners report they are easy to use, and do not have to remain flat on a tabletop, as do some other models.

➤ **Bayer Dex Glucometer** (called **Esprit** outside the United States)

➤ **Accu-Check Advantage** (called **Accu-Soft** outside the United States) – this meter is favored because it uses test strips that sip up the blood sample by capillary action.

Test strips are also available in many styles. Dog owners recommend Comfort Curve strips that use use capillary action to collect the blood sample. It is unnecessary to drip the blood onto the strip as with many other styles. FastTake strips have a confirmation window that indicates when a sufficient sample has been obtained.

How to Perform Home Blood Glucose Testing

For home glucose testing to be as accurate as possible, the skin pricks must be done where the dog has little or no fur. There are various appropriate sites to do this including the lip, elbow callus and footpad. The general description of the home testing procedure will be followed by details explaining how to use the dog's lip, elbow callus, and footpad.

Be sure to carefully read the instructions that come with your meter. You will need to calibrate it prior to the first use. Select a well-lit, quiet area in which to practice, free from distractions of family members and other pets. Wash your hands before you begin.

Prepare the supplies. Unwrap the test strip and uncap the lancet. If you are going to use a lancet pen, load it now. Prepare several food treats. Place all within easy reach.

It is important to prepare testing supplies in advance as there is only limited time before the meter must read the blood sample. If the meter permits, partially insert the test strip into it just prior to performing the blood stick. The meter will either flash or beep, alerting you that it is ready for the blood sample.

Position the dog as needed. Offer him a food treat and let him know that another one is waiting for him after the procedure. Talk to him reassuringly. If necessary, massage and relax him. Rub or tap the test site with your fingers. This will help stimulate blood flow.

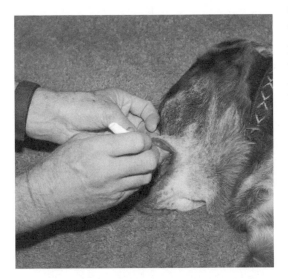

Gently pull the skin taut. It is easier to push the lancet into tissue that is taut. Quickly and firmly (almost forceful), push the lancet into the tissue. If using one of the lancet pens, first press it into the tissue and then fire it. Then relax the tension on the skin.

Squeeze or "milk" the area around the prick to help create a small droplet of blood. Avoid touching the actual prick site. Once the droplet has appeared, quickly bring the meter/test strip up to the drop of blood. The capillary action of the test strip will draw up the blood. Push the test strip completely into the machine. Reward the dog with food and lavish praise.

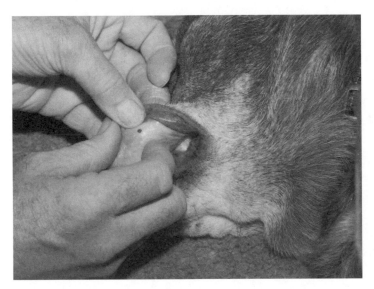

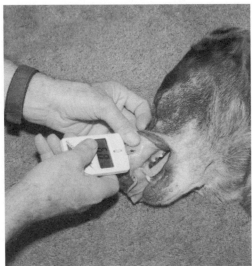

Lip Sticks: In the case of lip sticks, "lip" means one side or the other of the muzzle, not the actual lipline. Lip sticks may be performed with the dog lying down, standing, or sitting. When the dog lies on his side, blood flow will be improved. When the dog sits or stands, the dog owner can straddle the dog's back and hold him steady between his knees.

Inside of the Lip: This is the area most commonly used by dog owners. Slide the thumb or index finger of your nondominant hand under the dog's lip. Gently lift it upward and backward so that you can clearly see the inside of the lip. Avoid unnecessary pulling or pinching. Remove excess saliva with a quick wipe from a cloth, or by rubbing the inside lip with your

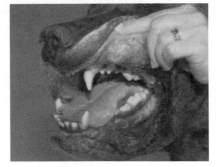

fingers several times. The latter will not only help dry the area, but also stimulate blood flow. Locate the area of the lip (not the gums) just above the canine tooth. There are many tiny blood vessels in this area. You may have better success pricking near the lip edge, but not on it.

Outside of the Lip: Slide the index finger of your nondominant hand under the dog's lip and gently pull it outward and toward you. Your middle finger and thumb will help keep the lip taut. The lip will essentially be wrapped around your index finger.

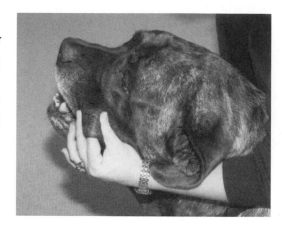

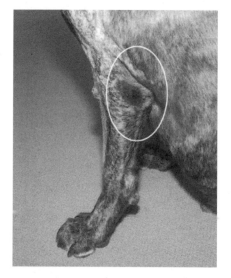

Callus Stick: Some dogs develop a callus behind the elbows of their front leg. It is an area where the coat wears away and the skin becomes thickened. It is more pronounced in large dogs and those with short coats. Not all dogs have elbow calluses. It may be helpful to have your dog stand for the callus stick. Gravity will aid blood flow to this area. Callused areas may require a larger lancet or more pressure on the lancet than will other sites.

Footpad stick: Other dog owners use either the footpad or the area just above it, in this approach. The latter option is a bit softer. Have the dog lie down for the footpad stick otherwise he may lose his balance. Lancet sites heal quickly and infection at the test site does not appear to be a problem.

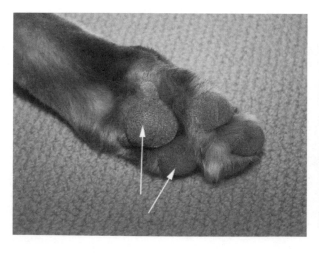

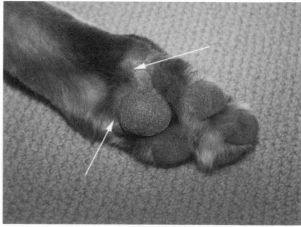

Helpful Hints for Home Blood Glucose Testing

If the aforementioned sites do not appeal to you, you may use the chin or shave a small area elsewhere on the body. Occasionally, a dog owner with medical training will draw blood from a vein.

If the prick site does not dry up immediately, apply a clean gauze or facial tissue to the area, and apply gentle pressure for about 60 seconds.

If you are having trouble obtaining a blood sample:

Apply a warm compress to area prior to the blood stick. This will help increase bloodflow. You can use a commercially available heating pad that is warmed in the microwave, or you can use a warm washcloth *inside* a plastic bag. (Moisture on the prick site can cause the blood drop to spread out instead of bead up.)

Prior to the test, smooth a thin layer of Vaseline over the area. Vaseline applied to dry areas (the callus, footpad, or outside of lip) can help the drop of blood bead up better. It can also help soften tough tissue like the callus or footpad. Vaseline may be less helpful on the inside of the lip.

If the blood droplet does not bead up, but rather disperses over the area (especially the inside of a wet lip), it can cause a low meter reading. Insufficient sample size (too little blood) is another common cause of a low reading.

Wait one second before milking the area. If you still do not see a good bead of blood wait two more seconds and squeeze again. Be patient. It may take a few moments for the blood drop to bead up.

Vascular anatomy (the position of blood vessels) differs from dog to dog and from one side of the body to the other. If you have difficulty getting a sufficient blood sample in one area, try another.

If you find it difficult to see whether you have performed a successful lancet prick, purchase a pair of magnifying reading glasses, a handheld magnifying glass, a headlamp (available at sporting good/camping stores), or a halogen reading lamp.

If you are having trouble with the equipment:

For example, if the meter (Glucometer Elite) runs out of time before you can get the blood sample, remove the test strip, wait a few moments, replace it, press the reset button, and continue.

You must get sufficient blood on the test strip in one attempt, rather than a little bit, and later a little bit more. Some meters will beep if you do not have a sufficient sample. Many strips have marks printed on them to indicate the volume needed.

If the reading is low, check the meter with the control solution. If it checks out adequately, repeat the test, ensuring that you collect an adequate sample. Offer your dog some Karo syrup or a snack if the low reading is repeated. Watch his behaviors closely. Take into consideration where your dog is in his normal glucose activity.

If you find the whole procedure overwhelming:

Put everything away for a few days. In the meantime, practice handling the dog's lips or paws during relaxed moments, such as when you watch TV. Offer him food treats during this time.

When a few days have passed, reread the procedure. It is common to forget information during moments of stress. Practice with the equipment and stuffed toy before trying again with the dog.

It is normal for first-time testers to be worried about "wounding" their pets. Most dog owners are more nervous about pricking their dog than the dog is about *being* pricked. Remember that the test sites on dogs are less sensitive than our fingers, the area human diabetics use to perform their tests. Finally, even experienced testers report that they, too, occasionally have trouble getting a good sample. It is easy to feel discouraged while learning this procedure. Stay optimistic!

Until you become adept at this procedure, it is likely that some of your readings may be slightly off due to inconsistent technique or procedure. Be certain that your technique is consistent before you and your veterinarian consider making a change in insulin dose.

When to Do Blood Testing (Spot Checks)

Many home-testers get in the habit of checking glucose levels before meals. Test your dog if he regurgitates a meal *after* you have given his insulin or whenever you recognize signs of hypoglycemia. Keep a log of your findings. These will help you and your veterinarian identify patterns in your dog's insulin activity.

When to Perform a Blood Glucose Curve

It is time to do a curve if you spot check your dog and the reading is low or shows a wide swing. One example would be a reading of 60 mg/dl in the morning and 300 mg/dl in the afternoon/evening.

You will need to choose a day when you will be home for 12 hours or more. Owners who wish to perform 24-hour curves set their alarm clock for 2-hour intervals through the night. Keep the dog's activity as routine as possible. Avoid extra treats, unusual amounts of exercise, and other stresses.

The first test should be performed *before* the morning meal and insulin injection. This is considered to be a baseline reading. If your dog is frantic to receive his breakfast, feed him first and follow immediately with the glucose test. The food will not be converted to glucose for an hour or more, so this reading should still be useful in evaluating baseline glucose levels. Repeat the reading at approximately 2-hour intervals. Greater intervals will not provide sufficient information.

Create a graph with blood glucose values along the left-hand side, and time of day going across the bottom. Plot your findings. As the dots accumulate, connect them with a line. The shape of the blood glucose curve will begin to appear. Contradictory to its name, the ideal blood glucose curve should be fairly flat, without wide swings.

Evaluating Blood Glucose Curves

Veterinarians use three important parameters to evaluate insulin activity. The first issue is **effectiveness of the insulin**. Naturally, the insulin should lower the blood glucose level, but it should also lower it to an acceptable range. For example, a drop from 180 mg/dl to 120 mg/dl is acceptable because the **nadir**, or lowest glucose level, falls within the scope of "being regulated." This is quite different than the same size drop (50 points) in a curve where the glucose drops from 350 mg/dl drops to 300 mg/dl. In this case, the lowest reading is still not within the scope of being regulated. (Ideally, the nadir should fall between 100 mg/dl and 125 mg/dl.) If there does not seem to be an effective drop in glucose levels, doctors consider *how much* **insulin** is being given.

Normally, dogs are dosed at a rate of 0.4 units of insulin per kilogram of body weight, but it is not unusual for individual dogs to need larger doses. If, however, a dog receives more than 2.2 units per kilogram, something may be contributing to insulin resistance or causing the dog difficulty in using insulin. This may include a concurrent disease, stress, infection or a female's heat cycle.

Consider again the curve that drops from 350 mg/dl to 300 mg/dl. If a dog is receiving a small dose of insulin (for example 0.6 U/kg), your veterinarian may recommend increasing the dose. If on the other hand, your dog is already receiving a large dose of insulin (2.2 U/kg) he may evaluate your dog for other health problems. The veterinarian may also wish to review your injection and storage techniques.

If the glucose curve demonstrates acceptable effectiveness and nadir, the doctor will then evaluate the **duration** of the insulin. This is defined as the period from injection time to when the blood glucose returns to 200 mg/dl or more. If a dog receives only one injection a day, it should, ideally, control blood glucose levels for the better part of a 24-hour period. In many cases, this does not occur and your veterinarian may switch your dog to a new type of insulin with 2 daily injections, each with a duration of approximately 12 hours. Reductions in dose often accompany such a switch. (Many dogs are prescribed 2 insulin injections at the time of diagnosis.)

It is important to note here, that *urine* glucose readings can differ dramatically from *blood* glucose readings taken at the same time. Additionally, blood glucose readings done at home differ from those done at the veterinary clinic. Different glucometers can provide different readings of the same blood sample. Veterinarians use blood samples drawn from a vein, whereas dog owners typically use capillary blood for their readings. Also, stress can increase blood glucose levels at the clinic. Remember to look for trends.

Making Changes in Insulin Dosages

This topic may represent one of the greatest concerns that veterinarians have with home glucose testing, i.e., that dog owners will inappropriately change doses without the veterinarian's knowledge or consent. Be sure to discuss questions you have about insulin adjustments with your veterinarian. As time passes, you will develop more expertise with this, and your veterinarian may give you guidelines for making adjustments by yourself.

Until that time, there are some guidelines that both you and perhaps your veterinarian may find helpful. Diabetic-dog owners have learned these points over the years — sometimes, the hard way.

It is best to initiate insulin changes on a day and at a time when you will be around to monitor your dog's behavior. Insulin changes are best made slowly and gradually. The most successful dosage changes are made by no more than 1/2 unit to 1 unit, per day. As the dog gets closer to being regulated, the veterinarian may have you increase by even smaller amounts.

Dogs should be evaluated for 3 days to 1 week after a change in dosage is made. This is the necessary time for a change in insulin to take effect, in most cases. Do *not* make adjustments on the basis of a single reading. Make insulin adjustments based on your discussions with your veterinarian and the help of a blood glucose curve. Doctors may also perform or recommend a blood glucose curve to assess the insulin activity at the new dose.

A flat graph of high numbers typically requires an increase in insulin. A wild curve with severe highs and lows suggests that the dog typically requires a *decrease* in insulin (see the following section on Somogyi Phenomenon). Many dog owners wait until they see a trend develop over several days before making any changes.

In cases where your dog refuses to eat, you will likely be instructed to skip the insulin injection altogether. Lack of appetite can also be a sign of *low* blood sugar (too much insulin). Discuss this possibility with your veterinarian. Appetite usually returns to normal once the insulin dose is reduced.

Making Changes in Mealtimes

As you learn more about your dog's diabetes and insulin activity, you may realize that small adjustments in his meals may help achieve better regulation. If a blood glucose curve demonstrates a severe drop in blood glucose, moving the mealtime closer to that point, or adding a snack, may minimize the drop.

In cases where free-feeding dogs are reaching high glucose levels when insulin activity is waning, it may be beneficial to limit access to food for those few hours. Discuss these options with your veterinarian.

Making Changes in Insulin Types

If your veterinarian switches your dog to a different type of insulin, he will likely reduce the dose as well. Individual dogs react differently to insulin, so undershooting the dose is done as a safety measure. This is especially important if the new insulin has a more potent action. Monitor your dog for signs of hypoglycemia when you administer a new type of insulin.

Difficulties in Getting Regulated

There are numerous reasons why a dog may be difficult to regulate. These reasons include problems with injection technique, the dog's general state of health, and insulin condition and dose.

Faulty injection technique is responsible for a great number of regulation problems. Review the technique covered in this chapter or demonstrate your technique to your veterinarian. Be certain that you are using the correct syringe for your strength of insulin (U-100 syringes with U-100 insulin, for example).

Some dog owners may be injecting insulin into the dog's skin instead of the SQ space. This results in slow uptake and action of the insulin. Other mistakes may include injection into the muscle or blood vessel. This would result in a premature uptake and action of the insulin.

The dog's general state of health can have an impact on regulation. Dehydration may adversely affect insulin activity. Recent steroid or dietary supplements can require an *increase* in insulin dose. The same is true for infections, inflammation, and the onset of such conditions as Cushing's disease and pancreatitis. Concurrent illness usually requires treatment before diabetic regulation can be achieved. Some dogs simply require what may seem to be an unusually large dose of insulin to become regulated.

Antibiotic use (eliminating an infection), changing diets (especially from commercial to homemade), and/or weight loss can result in *reduced* insulin need. The same is true for hormone (thyroid) use.

Another aspect of regulation is called "the honeymoon period." This phenomenon occurs more commonly in cats than it does in dogs. It earned its name because it occurs at the beginning cf the disease, just as a honeymoon occurs at the beginning of a marriage. Clinical signs include an intermittent need for insulin. It is believed that during the initial stages, some beta cells may still be periodically producing insulin before they are completely killed off.

Stress can also affect regulation. All of the following items can cause stress and raise blood glucose levels: a trip to the veterinary clinic or groomer (vaccinations or bathing); unusual activity, such as a trip to a dog show; an owner leaving for a trip; or having construction workers in your home.

Damaged or outdated insulin may also contribute to regulation difficulty. The type of insulin may simply not be the best choice for your pet. Discuss with your veterinarian options for switching to a type of insulin with a different action and duration or increasing to two injections per day, if not already doing so.

"Insulin resistance" is an often-misused term. True insulin resistance refers to the situation in which the body develops antibodies to insulin. This is a rare occurrence. More often, difficulty in getting a dog regulated is due to one of the aforementioned problems. A word of caution, however — overly aggressive insulin dosing can throw a diabetic dog into a complex rebound situation. It is known as the Somogyi Phenomenon, named after the doctor who identified it.

Somogyi is a confusing situation to most dog owners and many healthcare professionals, as well. Blood glucose levels drop low or suddenly and then rebound to extreme highs. It is an important concept to understand, and diabetic-dog owners, especially those performing home blood glucose testing, are encouraged to read the following section carefully.

The Somogyi Phenomenon

The Somogyi phenomenon describes another way in which the body protects itself from starvation. It occurs when the body receives more insulin than is needed and blood sugar drops extremely fast or low. The body perceives this as a sign of starvation and releases glucose previously stored in the liver into the bloodstream. Unfortunately, in the case of diabetics, the system causes more trouble than relief. In these dogs, the insulin injection wears off, just as the glucose is being released from the liver. These two events result in extremely high blood glucose levels, commonly 300 mg/dl or more.

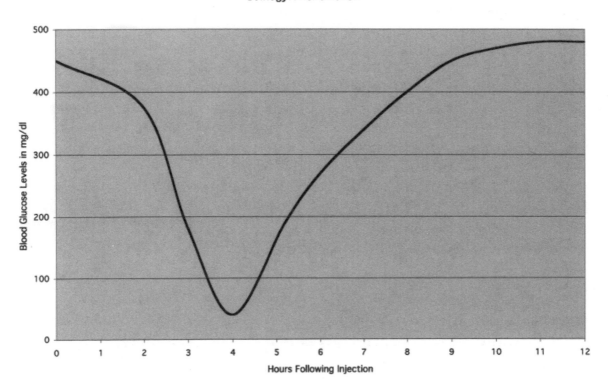

Somogyi Phenomenon

The natural (but incorrect) inclination is to increase the next insulin dosage. This begins a vicious cycle. The increase in insulin quickly and drastically reduces glucose levels. The body reacts by again releasing stored glucose into the bloodstream. And the result is a repeated rebound in glucose (high readings) as the insulin activity wears off.

You may sometimes hear the phenomena referred to as rebound hyperglycemia, insulin induced hyperglycemia, or hypoglycemic induced hyperglycemia. Whatever the terminology, it is a case of high blood glucose levels that *result from too much insulin*.

Somogyi can occur anytime there is excess insulin — when dosages are changed too quickly; when a new, more potent insulin is prescribed; or when there is an overlap of activity from one injection to another. Dog owners frequently (and unwittingly) start the Somogyi cycle when they increase insulin dosages based on high spot-test readings. If you are giving your dog increasingly higher doses of insulin and he *continues* to experience signs of polydipsia, polyuria, or high blood glucose levels, it is very possible you have exceeded his ideal dose and are witnessing the Somogyi effect.

During the Somogyi phenomena, dog owners tend to be most concerned with the high glucose numbers. The real danger, however, lies in the possibility of severe hypoglycemic attack. If you were doing urine glucose testing on a dog in Somogyi, you would most likely notice high readings on the morning test.

Once you and your veterinarian have identified that Somogyi is in effect, you will likely be instructed to reduce the dog's insulin by 10% to 25%. If the Somogyi swings have been especially severe, you may be instructed to return to the last dosage at which the dog was regulated.

After 3 days to a week, the Somoygi effect should resolve itself. Your veterinarian may have you slowly begin increasing the dose by 1/2 to 1 unit per day, once every three days or so. This will likely be followed up with another blood glucose curve. Suspending all insulin is usually not recommended.

It may take several days for a dog to return to normal following a Somogyi episode. Dogs appear to be somewhat resistant to the effects of insulin for about 72 hours afterwards. Blood glucose curves done immediately afterward are not helpful as they demonstrate exaggerated readings. Avoid future episodes by reducing sharp lows in the daily glucose curve.

Additional Tests to Monitor Glucose Control

In addition to measuring urine glucose and blood glucose, there are two more laboratory tests your veterinarian may use to evaluate glucose control. These tests include the **fructosamine test** and the **glycosylated hemoglobin test.**

When glucose circulates in the bloodstream, it binds with protein molecules that are also present. The protein is then termed "glycosylated." One such protein is hemoglobin (the protein in red blood cells). Other such proteins include serum albumins.

Each of these proteins has a fairly consistent life span. Hemoglobin has a life span of about 3 to 4 months. Serum albumin has a life span of about 1 to 3 weeks. It is possible to measure how many proteins have become glycosylated when a blood sample is collected.

The fructosamine test measures how many glucose-albumin molecules are present. This demonstrates how much glucose, on average, has been present in the bloodstream during the past 1 to 3 weeks. The glycosylated hemoblobin test measures glucose averages over the past few months (as opposed to weeks). Of the two tests, the fructosamine test is more commonly performed on dogs.

These tests can be of value in confirming that a dog is reasonably well-regulated. However, since the reading is *an average* of extreme highs and lows, even a poorly-regulated dog can have an acceptable reading on a fructosamine test. To illustrate specific patterns in insulin activity and glucose control, a blood glucose curve should be performed.

Ketoacidosis

Finally, in our discussion of diabetic regulation, we come to the topic of ketoacidosis, the result of uncontrolled diabetes. Ketoacidosis occurs when there is insufficient insulin to help glucose into the cells. In such cases, the body secretes cortisol to break down muscle tissue and body fat into glucose. This protective mechanism, known as catabolism or lypolysis, attempts to feed starving cells.

The byproducts of these processes are ketone acids or, simply, ketones. Ketone acids are eliminated from the body through the urine and pulmonary activity (breathing). Urinary output increases to flush them out. As these waste products build up, they can be measured in the urine. The increased urination can cause severe dehydration and alter the body's metabolic balance.

Signs of ketoacidosis include many of the signs previously discussed, such as polydipsia, polyuria, weakness, vomiting, and lethargy. There are a few more specific signs, as well. These include dehydration, ketonuria (ketones present in the urine), and a sweet, fruity fragrance to the breath. The latter is not as reliable a measure as ketoacidosis, however.

Your veterinarian may encourage you to measure your dog's urine for the presence of ketones, especially when first becoming regulated, or when your dog experiences a concurrent illness. Urine test strips are available to test for ketones alone (Ketostix) or for ketones in combination with glucose (Keto-Diastix.) If ketones are present, immediately report this to your vet. He will likely instruct you to increase the insulin dosage, and by what amount.

If left untreated, ketoacidosis can progress to a life-threatening stage. Dogs that are severely ketoacidotic require hospitalization for intravenous hydration, short acting (R) insulin to quickly transport glucose into the cells, electrolytes supplements, and continuing blood work.

Exercise and the Diabetic Dog

A diagnosis of diabetes does not mean the end of physical activity for your dog. On the contrary, exercise helps reduce stress and obesity and improves insulin action. If your dog was active and relatively healthy before the diabetes, he can continue these activities. Many diabetic dogs continue to play hours of fetch, take long walks, and swim. As a dog's diabetes becomes regulated and he feels better, he may begin to increase his activity on his own.

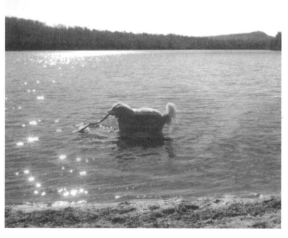

Photo courtesy of Pam Lardear

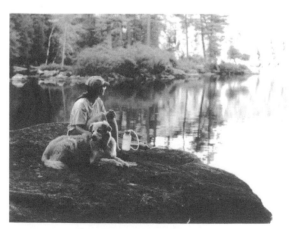

Photo courtesy of Garrie Stevens

There are, however, some safety precautions to keep in mind. Exercise causes the body to metabolize insulin and glucose at a faster rate. Unexpected or extended periods of exercise can cause difficulty in getting a dog initially regulated. Hypoglycemia can result if the exercise occurs at the same time insulin activity peaks. *Hyperg*lycemia can result if the exercise occurs at the same time insulin activity (duration) wanes. In this case, the exercise will cause quick metabolism of whatever insulin *is* available, leaving excess glucose in the blood. This is another example of why it is important to understand your dog's insulin activity.

There are several ways to minimize the chances of a hypoglycemic event. First, try to maintain some level of consistency in activity from day to day. This includes days when *your* schedule changes, too. For example, if you enjoy taking your dog on a short hike on weekends, try to take a similar walk each weekday, as well. Consistency, timing, and moderation are key elements.

Exercise is best had a few hours after meals, *after* the insulin activity has peaked but *before* the end of the insulin activity. This will help avoid extreme highs and lows in blood glucose. If you perform home blood glucose testing, test his blood before and/or after you embark on unexpected activity. If his blood is in the range of normal or slightly low, offer him a snack.

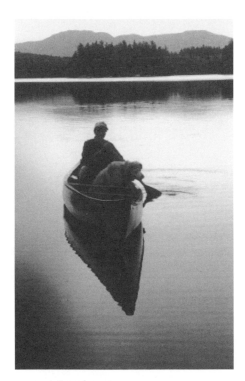

Photo courtesy of Garrie Stevens

Traveling With a Diabetic Dog

When traveling with a diabetic dog, be certain to bring all the supplies you normally use and back up supplies, as well. Bring sufficient food and supplements, such as dietary enzymes. Keep the insulin bottle in a cooler, but avoid direct contact with ice as this could damage the insulin. Be certain to bring Karo or pancake syrup and the phone number for your vet or emergency clinic.

Some dog owners tape an informational card on the dog's crate or the dashboard. This can include insulin instructions and emergency phone numbers. If you are traveling across time zones, make changes toward the new time schedule gradually. (See page 79.)

Traveling Without Your Dog

If you must leave your dog behind when you travel, there are several options available to you. You may enlist the services of a qualified dog-sitter. Some services visit the dog several times daily. If you have a trusted friend, neighbor, or veterinary technician, you may be able to secure their services overnight, as well.

You will need to train the pet-sitter in diabetic care if he is unfamiliar with it. Have him demonstrate his injection technique before you leave. Write out instructions that deal with emergency situations.

If having a house-sitter is not an option, you may board your dog at a commercial boarding kennel or veterinary clinic. The latter option does offer an added measure of safety, especially if the clinic is staffed 24 hours a day. Write out instructions as to his insulin doses, feeding, and exercise. If the kennel will feed homemade food, bring ample supplies.

Kenneling a dog is not without drawbacks, however. It can be very stressful for the dog, which may significantly raise blood glucose levels. The kennel may not feed homemade food, even though you make the effort to provide it. Many kennels have antiquated regulations that require excessive vaccinations. This is contraindicated in pets that have immune system disorders. ✳

Chapter 10

Caring for Dogs With Cushing's Disease and Excess Cortisol Production

The type of treatment prescribed for Hyperadrenocorticism (HAC) is largely dependent upon the cause — whether it is pituitary-dependent, adrenal-dependent, or iatrogenic (caused by prescription steroid use). In cases of iatrogenic HAC, eliminating prescription steroids will often return cortisol levels to normal. Prescription steroids must be withdrawn slowly, over several weeks, to give the adrenal glands ample time to resume cortisol production. Normal adrenal function usually returns over the course of several months.

Surgical Treatment

Adrenal gland tumors are sometimes removed surgically, based on the nature of the tumor. *Benign* adrenal tumors may be excised by removing the entire adrenal gland (adrenalectomy), but the risks associated with this procedure are high. Postoperative complications are common, as the dog's immune system is compromised. Seek the services of a board-certified specialist for this procedure. Dogs will require a lifetime of cortisol replacement therapy postoperatively.

Pituitary gland tumors are *not* surgically removed. They are treated medically and sometimes with radiation therapy. There are three medications commonly prescribed at present: Lysodren, the traditional therapy; Anipryl, a medication used in Canada, and only recently available in the United States; and less commonly, Ketoconazole (or Nizoral).

Medical Treatment

Through different means, the following drugs reduce the production of cortisol. They are often prescribed "to effect" or "to tolerance." That is, they are dosed until the dog demonstrates signs of cortisol levels falling to, or *below,* normal. The latter scenario is described as *hypo*adrenocorticism, or Addison's disease. Signs include vomiting, diarrhea, weakness, lack of appetite, and depression. If your dog exhibits any of these signs, alert your veterinarian or emergency veterinary clinic immediately.

Conditions such as arthritis, allergies, and autoimmune diseases can be masked during periods of excess cortisol production. Once cortisol levels are controlled, it is not uncommon for these conditions to express themselves. In such cases, it may be helpful to reduce the irritating factors found in most commercial diets, in an attempt to balance inflammatory reactions and steroid production.

Lysodren

The drug Lysodren (also known as Mitotane or o,p'-DDD) is a powerful medication that was originally developed as a chemotherapy drug but is also useful in cases of HAC. It destroys the cortisol-producing layer of the adrenal gland. It can be used both in cases of adrenal-dependent *and* pituitary-dependent HAC.

Therapy is begun with a period known as the induction or loading phase. During this period of 1 to 8 weeks, the dog receives a daily dose of Lysodren to bring cortisol production under control. A typical dose is 50mg per kilogram of body weight, per day. (Divide pounds by a factor of 2.2 to get a measurement in kilograms.) Most loading phases last between 7 and 10 days. Some dogs may be hospitalized during this time, but most are treated at home. Clinical signs of the disease are often improved within just a few days.

Your veterinarian may ask you to monitor water consumption for a 24-hour period prior to the induction phase. To monitor water intake, mark the inside of the dog's water bowl with a waterproof marking pen, denoting cups, 1/2 cups, 1/4 cups, or even ounces, for small dogs. Keep written records in a small journal or on the calendar. This method may be more reliable than trying to monitor urine output, since a dog with free access to the yard may urinate when you are not watching.

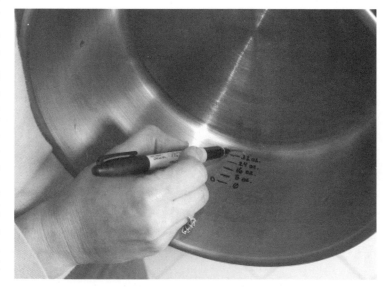

Average daily water consumption is approximately 1 cup of water for every 10 pounds of body weight (or 250 ml for every 4.5 kg of body weight). Dogs eating homemade diets typically drink less. If you have more than one dog, they may need to be separated during the time you are trying to monitor water intake, each with his own water source.

You must also monitor your dog daily for any signs of listlessness or loss of appetite. These signs indicate that cortisol levels have dropped sufficiently. If all family members are away from home during the day, consider having a trusted neighbor check the dog's condition.

Lysodren is a powerful medication and it is common for dogs to experience a number of other reactions during induction. These can include muscle weakness (especially in the rear legs), liver complications, stomach upset, vomiting, and loss of coordination. Dividing the dose over several days may help reduce the severity of side effects. Some adverse reactions are even more serious. A small percentage of dogs may experience fast-growing pituitary tumors during induction. This is caused by the rapid decrease in cortisol levels, which in turn, raises ACTH levels, stimulates the pituitary gland, and results in tumor growth.

In dogs that produce biologically inactive cortisol, or in those with exhausted adrenal function, Lysodren use can prove fatal. It destroys the small amount of adrenal tissue that is still functioning. If not closely monitored, these dogs can suddenly crash in a severe episode of Addison's disease. Remember that a certain level of cortisol is necessary for life.

Oral prednisone is often prescribed in combination with Lysodren in an attempt to minimize side effects. This allows for a slow and steady withdrawal of cortisol from the system. Keep in mind that prednisone may cause blood glucose levels to fluctuate, especially in the diabetic.

An ACTH test may be performed 7 to 10 days after the loading dose. This will indicate whether cortisol levels are within acceptable limits. The goal is to achieve a resting (pre-test) cortisol level between 1-5 ug/dl (U.S.) or 30-110 mmol/l (Canada) and a post-test level that does not rise much higher than this. This is called a flatline or "blunted" response. When this goal is reached, it is considered to be the end of the loading phase, and the beginning of the maintenance phase.

Maintenance therapy involves a smaller dose of medication prescribed long-term (50mg per kg, per *week*). Unless your dog experiences gastrointestinal upset, he will likely receive medication once a week. Medication should be given with meals. Long-term therapy is necessary because the adrenal glands can regenerate and return to their previous levels of cortisol production. It is not uncommon for Cushinoid dogs to become unregulated and require repeated loading doses within the first 12 months. Cases of adrenal-dependent HAC may require higher doses than pituitary-dependent cases.

Periodic rechecks are necessary. This is usually accomplished by ACTH tests at 3- to 6-month periods. Follow-up is an important part of treatment as overdose is a realistic threat. Should overdose and Addison's disease result, a dog is medicated with oral prednisone to replace the total loss of adrenal function.

Anipryl

Anipryl (also known as L-Deprenyl, Eldepryl, or Selegiline) is a medication humans use to control Parkinson's disease. It is used in dogs to control signs of canine cognitive dysfunction (senility) and more recently, to control *pituitary-dependent* HAC in some countries. It is ineffective in cases of adrenal-dependent disease. Anipryl is considered to be less toxic than Lysodren, and some veterinarians consider it a good choice for uncomplicated cases of Cushing's disease diagnosed early on.

Anipryl works by increasing levels of dopamine, a hormone in the brain. Increased levels of dopamine are believed to decrease ACTH production. Treatment does not require a loading phase. Instead, dogs are usually placed on medication for a two-month period. If signs of the disease have not been controlled during that time (which is common), the dose will likely be increased. If this continues to prove ineffective, your dog may be tested for concurrent illness or switched to Lysodren. Follow-up ACTH testing is not applicable, since Anipryl only works on dopamine levels, not pituitary or adrenal function.

Anipryl can also cause certain adverse reactions (including diarrhea and vomiting), but they are fewer than those caused by Lysodren. Anipryl can have a different type of drawback, however. It is unsuccessful in the majority of cases.

Many dog owners complain that it is ineffective, other than at very high doses. They become frustrated by the prolonged period of unregulated Cushing's disease. This is understandable, since the dog may experience continued systemic damage from high cortisol levels, incontinence, hunger, depression, and weakness during this time.

Ketaconazole

This is an antifungal medication that, through a side effect, reduces levels of cortisol. It does this by inhibiting enzyme reactions that normally result in the release of adrenal cortisol. It must be administered every 12 hours and can be expensive. It is prescribed less commonly than either of the previously mentioned drugs. As with Lysodren, Ketaconazole requires a loading phase and periodic ACTH tests to check effectiveness.

Dietary Therapy

Dietary therapy can be an additional and realistic option for treating symptoms of excess cortisol production, especially when a formal diagnosis of Cushing's Disease has not been made. Therapy can include a homemade diet void of grain products and supplements such as Phosphatydl Serine. (See Chapter 8, *Dietary Management.*)

Comfort Measures

In addition to medical and surgical treatments, there are a variety of measures the dog owner can implement to make a Cushinoid dog more comfortable.

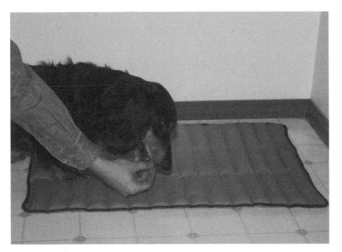

Heat Intolerance

Until cortisol levels are controlled, help your dog manage signs of heat intolerance by offering him a cool place to rest. This can be a small plastic pool in the yard, frozen water bottles in his crate, or cooling pads in the house. Cooling pads are available commercially or can be homemade. Some contain polymer crystals that are soaked in water.

Some pads are *filled* with water or other coolants. (One owner placed dry, frozen, soup beans inside a pillowcase.) This style may be more attractive to some dogs since the pads are cool but still dry to the touch. (See Supplier's section.) These pads may also be more attractive to owners since they can be placed on wall-to-wall carpeting without causing damage.

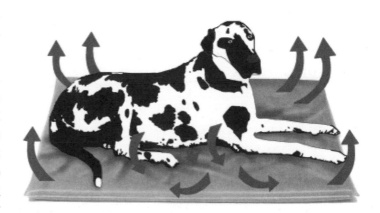

Photo courtesy of Maverick Marketing

If you can sew, you can make your own cooling pad with heavy cotton fabric and polymer granules available at plant nurseries. These granules absorb enormous amounts of water.

Instructions:

Cut the fabric to the size pad appropriate for your dog. Sew around three sides. Sew parallel tubes about 1.5 inches wide. Place approximately 1 teaspoon of granules for each 12 inches of tube length. Then sew across the fourth side of the mat, closing off all the tubes. Soak the pad in cool water for about 30 minutes. Refrigerate the mat when it becomes too warm. Completely dry the mat if you need to remove or add more crystals.

Even though your dog will eventually appreciate the cooling pad, he may be reluctant to use it at first. Introduce your dog to the cooling pad with food treats. Do not force him onto the pad. First, feed him near the pad. Later, place treats on the pad. If he places a foot on it, reward him with praise and additional treats. As you repeat this experience, the dog will come to view the pad as a positive thing. He will become less apprehensive and eventually begin to use it.

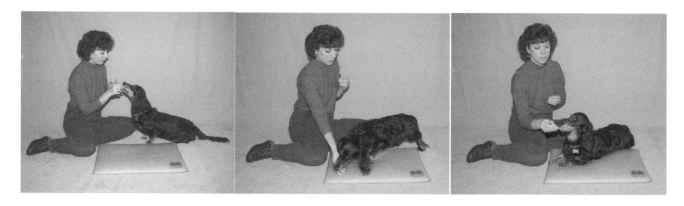

Muscle Weakness

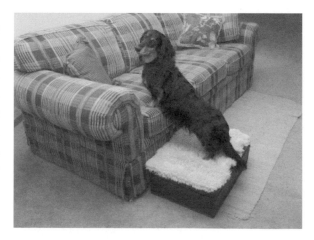

Many dog owners implement the use of ramps and footstools for their dogs with muscle weakness. Footstools can be used to help a dog make the transition from floor to furniture, and vice versa. (The footstool pictured at right is actually a small wicker chest covered with a bath mat.) Ramps can also be used in such situations, as well as for access to automobiles and to negotiate partial flights of stairs.

If you pursue such an option, enlist the skills of an experienced carpenter or builder (or see "Suppliers" list). It would be detrimental to the dog's self-confidence to have a ramp collapse or slip out from under him. Tack down anti-skid tape such as that found on commercial building stairways or outdoor carpeting. Consider building a wall or safety railing to keep the dog from inadvertently walking off the side of the ramp. The longer the flight of stairs, the longer the ramp must be.

Introduce your dog to the ramp with a food treat held close to his nose. If he is reluctant to step onto the ramp, dab on bits of peanut butter, cream cheese, or other soft food treat up the ramp in a row. (Kibble, after all, would roll to the bottom!) Offer him verbal encouragement to find each succeeding treat.

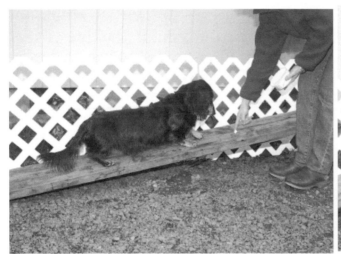 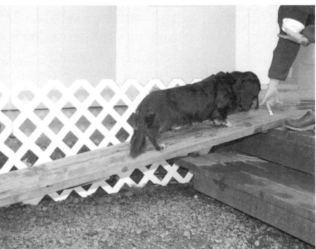

If you have wooden, tile, or linoleum floor coverings, consider laying out rubber mats or carpet runners with rubber backing. A variety of these are commercially available at home-improvement stores, carpet stores, and some hardware stores. They can be cut in half width wise to accommodate small dogs and be cost-effective.

Place an additional mat under the dog's food bowl. This will offer him extra security during mealtime. You can also provide your dog with raised food and water bowls, which may contribute to steadiness on his feet.

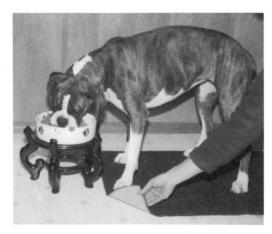

Assist large, weak, or unsteady dogs down the stairs by slipping a towel under their belly to serve as a sling. You can also use a canvas log-carrier (the type found at fireplace shops), as they often are constructed with handles. These techniques can also help weak dogs manage slick floors at the veterinary clinic or grooming shop.

Finally, purchase socks designed for human babies or specially designed dog socks for walking dogs outdoors in snow or ice. These are designed with rubber gripper soles or strips.

Trouble With Medications

If your dog is prescribed a small dose of medication, you may be required to split the pills, which may be difficult to accomplish with an ordinary kitchen knife. Ask you pharmacist for information on pill-cutters, small plastic gadgets that cleanly and evenly divide tablets. Handle Lysodren pills as little as possible. Wear latex gloves when you handle pills, or wash your hands afterward. Lysodren is a powerful medication that may carry exposure risks to humans.

If your dog experiences stomach upset from his Cushing's medications, discuss with your veterinarian the option of giving a nonprescription antacid, such as Pepcid AC. Remember to give medication with meals or even 30 to 40 minutes afterward. If all else fails, discuss the option of dividing the dose between several days. ✳

Chapter 11

Caring for Dogs With Pancreatic Disease

Treatment of acute and chronic pancreatitis may differ, but the goals of both remain the same — including resting the pancreas, reducing its workload, and minimizing complications such as inflammation, pain, and dehydration. Pancreatic enzyme insufficiency is primarily treated with enzyme replacements.

Treating Acute Pancreatitis

Most cases of acute pancreatitis will resolve in a few days when the GI tract is allowed to rest. This is accomplished by withholding food and water from the dog for 3 to 5 days. During this time, necessary fluids are supplied to the dog by intravenous (IV) infusion. Dogs receiving IV fluids may be kept in the veterinary hospital or may return several times daily for new fluids.

After several days, blood enzyme levels will be retested. When these levels return to normal or near-normal levels, your veterinarian will likely offer the dog a drink of water. If no vomiting occurs in the next 12 to 24 hours, your veterinarian will offer food in small amounts. Dogs are typically sent home when they are eating and drinking normally.

In concurrent cases of acute pancreatitis and diabetes mellitus, veterinarians may recommend total parenteral nutrition (TPN), a method of providing liquid nutrition. A plastic/silicone tube is passed into the dog's stomach and a liquid formula is slowly injected through the tube several times daily.

Since TPN only provides a fraction of the normal calories, your veterinarian will decrease insulin dosages accordingly. As the pancreatitis resolves, insulin dosages will gradually be increased as the dog returns to his normal intake. This may take several weeks. Bouts of pancreatitis may cause a diabetic dog to experience insulin resistance at a later time.

Other aspects of treatment may include anti-emetic medications prescribed for severe vomiting, painkillers to reduce abdominal discomfort, and antibiotics to prevent bacterial infection. Surgery may be indicated in cases of pancreatic cysts or abscesses. Sadly, even with diligent care and treatment, some cases of acute pancreatitis may still prove fatal.

Treating Chronic Pancreatitis

Cases of chronic pancreatitis are most often approached through dietary treatment. Many veterinarians agree that easily digestible diets are helpful to chronic pancreatitis. In reviewing Chapter 7, it is clear that highly processed, grain-based diets are *not* easily digested by the dog. Canine nutritionists recommend feeding a diet containing lean meats and 50% or more of pulped vegetables. They recommend avoiding grain and dairy products in the diet and supplementing cooked diets with digestive enzymes.

Digestive enzymes are made from pancreatin, a synthetic product extracted from bovine sources, or plant sources. Prescription brands and those prepared from animal sources are typically more concentrated than are those available over the counter. Certain holistic supply houses now offer stronger preparations available to the public. (See Suppliers section.)

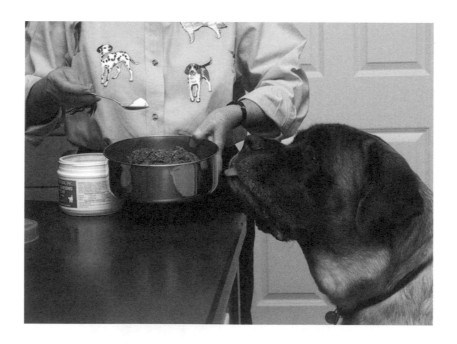

Most of these preparations are offered in a powdered form that is sprinkled on the dog's food. Tablets are also available. These may be more cost-effective, but they may be more labor-intensive, as well, since tablets must be crushed to work well.

Treating Pancreatic Enzyme Insufficiency (PEI)

PEI is also treated by the addition of digestive enzymes to the diet. This is usually enough to control the signs of PEI, but in difficult cases, antacids are sometimes prescribed to reduce the effects of hydrochloric acid. This contributes to improved enzyme function.

Anti-diarrhea agents may also be prescribed. Use a large syringe or turkey baster to administer oral anti-diarrhea medications, such as Kaopectate or Pepto-Bismol. Place the tip in the back corner of the dog's mouth and inject slowly so the medication does not choke him. If your dog is prone to shake his head when wet, administer the medication outdoors or you may find it all over your walls as well. Some of these medications are also available in tablet form.

Another concern with PEI is bacterial overgrowth in the intestine. While certain types and amounts of bacteria are normal in the GI tract, stressed intestinal tissue may become host to foreign bacteria. This overgrowth, combined with chronic irritation, may hamper the work of dietary enzyme supplements. Lactobacillus Acidophilus, one of the normal and friendly bacteria, can be supplied by yogurt or special dietary supplements called probiotics. By furnishing friendly bacteria, you reduce the chances of colonization by foreign types. ✳

Chapter 12

Additional Health Concerns

There are number of additional health concerns that may affect your dog. Some are a result of high cortisol levels, some are related to the dog's compromised immune system, and others are a result of the high levels of chemicals found in commercial diets. They frequently occur in combination, since the dog's entire immune/digestive/endocrine system is stressed.

In many cases, prevention is the best medicine. You may not be able to forestall these health problems, but catching them in their early stages can be beneficial to your dog. The first step in this process is to perform frequent physical assessments. This involves a head-to-toe examination of your dog to check for signs of infection, injury, or changes in tissue or coat.

Physical Assessment

Begin by examining your dog's head. Look inside his ears, mouth, and at his teeth and gums. Signs of infection can include swelling, unpleasant odor, or discharge. Examine his eyes. Check for cloudiness or discharge. Gently lift the upper eyelid and check that the "whites of his eyes" are white, not red. Remain alert for vision loss in his daily activities.

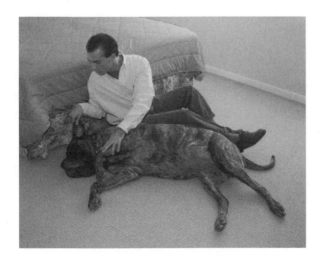 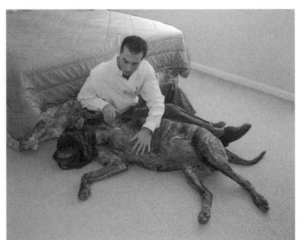

Run your hands over his head, through his fur, and down his neck. Check for any injuries, lacerations, bumps, and lumps. Run your hands along his back, his chest, and each side of his body. Check each leg and the pads of his feet. Gently spread apart his toes. Check for irritation (redness) or yeasty skin infection (often accompanied by redness or brown discharge). Check between your dog's hind legs and around his tail. The skin fold between the thighs is a common location for skin irritations to develop. Urinary tract infections can cause redness, swelling, discharge, and dribbling urine.

Complete an assessment several times each week. Choose a time when the dog is relaxed. It is a pleasurable activity for most dogs and their owners. Report changes or unusual findings to your veterinarian.

Other Preventive Measures

If your dog continues to experience frequent infections, incontinence, or gastrointestinal problems, consider or reconsider switching your dog to a home-made diet, if you have not already done so. It may not eliminate all complications, but it may help reduce the frequency and severity of symptoms.

Infections

Several factors contribute to the high incidence of infections in diabetic, Cushinoid, and sub-Cushinoid dogs. They include depressed immune system function (white blood cell activity) and a high-sugar environment (conducive to bacterial growth). Yeast is a common cause of infections. It, too, thrives on excess sugar and reproduces quickly in moist conditions. Some dog owners describe the dark brown discharge of yeast infection as "the creeping crud."

Infections can result in a vicious cycle. They raise blood glucose levels and cause difficulty in keeping a diabetic dog regulated. Long-term prescription steroids further stress the immune system and hormonal function. This contributes to additional difficulty regulating blood sugar and greater chance for infection.

In most cases of infection, oral antibiotics will be prescribed for your dog. It is crucial that your dog complete the entire course of medication, even if signs appear to subside. If a dog is only medicated for a few days, the bacteria can become *stronger* and more resistant to drug treatment in the future. Antibiotics may be prescribed for few weeks, a month, or even longer periods in severe cases.

If your veterinarian does prescribe antibiotics, consider adding the beneficial bacteria, acidophilus (available in yogurt or powder form) to your dog's diet. Antibiotics kill beneficial bacteria in the intestine, and adding acidophilus prevents the overgrowth of more aggressive bacteria. You may also find specific preparations known as probiotic powders. These include a combination of several beneficial bacteria and are available from veterinarians or pet supply stores. (See Supplier's section.)

Skin Infections

Yeast and fungal growth can occur between toes, around the face, and at the ends of long ears. If in doubt, your veterinarian can do a scraping to diagnose the problem. Common signs of skin infection include itching, licking (especially of the paws), a dark greasy discharge, and possible hair loss.

Help prevent yeast infections by minimizing damp environments. Be sure to dry off wet feet when the dog comes in from the rain or snow. Clip long hair around feet so they dry faster. Wipe beards and faces dry after a drink in the water bowl. Purchase special bowls (tall, thin, and bucket-shaped) that keep long ears from getting wet. (See Supplier's section.)

Apply an antifungal powder (often available from your veterinarian or over the counter at your local pharmacy) in between toes and skin folds. Your vet will likely prescribe oral or topical antibiotics and possibly a medicated shampoo, as well.

Ear Infections

Yeast and bacteria growth inside the ears can produce a dark greasy discharge with an unpleasant odor. Common signs include scratching and head-shaking behaviors. Occasionally, infection and scarring can cause deafness or equilibrium problems.

It is important to keep the ear canal clean. Your veterinarian may prescribe a cleansing and drying solution to use inside the ears, as well as oral antibiotics and topical steroids. These infections can be very tenacious and difficult to cure.

Oral Infections and Complications

Gingivitis, considered by some to be another autoimmune disease, commonly occurs along with diabetes. Dental plaque is a frequent finding in dogs that eatcommercial diets. Excess cortisol can cause pain and weakness in the ligament of the mouth and gums.

Ask your veterinarian to show you how to brush your dog's teeth and gums. There are special toothbrush kits designed just for pets. Also consider the benefits of allowing your dog to eat fresh foods.

Urinary Tract Infections (UTIs)

UTIs can involve several structures, including the kidneys, but most often refer to infections of the bladder. Several factors contribute to bladder infections. These can include glucosuria (glucose in the urine), depressed white blood cell function, immunoglobulin A (IgA) deficiency, and the high levels of impurities (chemicals and poor quality protein) present in commercial diets. The latter irritate and inflame the bladder lining much as they inflame the intestinal lining. This inflammation primes the bladder for infection.

Signs of UTIs can include frequent licking of the urethra, incontinence or dribbling of urine, blood in the urine, straining, urgency (frequently asking to go outside) without being able to produce much volume, increased thirst, and lethargy.

To diagnose a bladder infection, your veterinarian may request that you collect a urine sample and deliver it to the clinic. There are several ways to collect a urine sample. The sample does not need to be sterile for this examination, only clean. You can use a clean ceramic mug, margarine container, or plastic zip-style bag.

Follow the dog into the yard. Walk along with him, but pretend you are not very interested in his activities. Most dogs are accustomed to relieving themselves, *by* themselves, and may be intimidated if their owner follows them around. After the dog squats or lifts his leg, quietly slip the cup or container under the urine stream, once he has started. If he seems especially alarmed by what you are doing, offer him a food treat afterward.

If your aim is poor, and the idea of urine on your hand bothers you, purchase a pair or box of latex gloves. You may also use a clean pooper-scooper or soup ladle to catch the urine, transferring it to a small container afterward. This alleviates the need to bend down.

It is best to bring a fresh urine sample (within an hour of being collected) to your veterinarian. If this is not possible, refrigerate the urine sample until it is time to leave for the clinic. This will help prevent excess bacteria from growing in the sample, which might skew the findings.

In more difficult UTI cases, your veterinarian may obtain a sterile sample by performing Urine is collected through a sterile needle inserted through the skin, directly into the bladder. This can provide a more accurate urine sample when there is difficulty identifying or treating infectious agents.

Your veterinarian may encourage you to add acidic fruit or supplements to your dog's diet: cranberries, blueberries, cranberry supplement, or Azocran tablets. All of these acidify the urine, which helps to discourage bacterial growth.

You can monitor urine acidity by measuring urine pH levels. This is performed with pH urine test strips, much in the manner that home urine testing is performed. Urine pH strips are available at your local pharmacy.

Keep your dog well hydrated. The more frequently a dog empties his bladder, the less chance bacterial infection has to get started. Add some type of flavoring to the dog's drinking water, such as soy sauce or soup bouillon. If your dog has sodium restrictions, purchase low-sodium types. Discuss your plans with your veterinarian.

Remember that UTIs can cause a vicious cycle. The infection causes higher blood sugar levels that, in turn, cause excess sugar to spill into the bladder. This sets the stage for even more bacterial growth. Discuss the need for better blood glucose control with your veterinarian.

Dietary Management of Infection

Canine nutritionists recommend treating chronic infections from the inside of the body, outward. In addition to whatever treatments your veterinarian prescribes, nutritionists recommend acidifying the dog's system through dietary means. If you are feeding a homemade food, remove any grain and high-sugar fruits and vegetables from the diet. This includes bananas, apples, sweet potatoes, yams, carrots, green peas, corn, parsnips, winter squash, and tomatoes.

Commercial dog food, especially kibble, is very alkaline. If you continue to feed commercial food, acidify the system by adding vitamin C, *raw* apple cider vinegar (available at health food stores, not grocery stores), and cranberry juice or cranberry extract, or frozen blueberries. In addition, some research indicates that *highly bio-available protein* (homemade diets with raw *or* cooked meat) discourages bacteria from developing in the urinary tract.

Renal (Kidney) Problems

Kidney Infection

Frequent or long-term, low-grade bladder infections can travel into the kidneys. Signs of kidney infection can include dilute urine, blood in the urine, vomiting, and decreased appetite. These, like bladder infections, are treated with potent, sometimes long-term antibiotics.

Kidney Degeneration

Separate from kidney infection, is the case of kidney degeneration, the gradual loss of kidney function. Signs can include dilute urine, dehydration, and electrolyte imbalance. Polyuria is the primary cause of magnesium deficiency. Kidneys that are scarred from dietary impurities and function poorly, can not filter excess phosphorus from the bloodstream. When phosphorus accumulates, the body pulls calcium from the bones to bind the phosphorus and carry it away. This is another way in which high levels of calcium become present in the blood stream and soft tissues of the body. Clinical signs can include joint pain, lameness, and itchiness. Chronic kidney degeneration can also result in anemia, weakness and loss of appetite.

Two schools of thought exist as to how best to deal with kidney disease. Most veterinarians prescribe specially formulated, low-protein, low-phosphorous commercial diets. They believe these will minimize uremic toxins and slow down renal failure. Advanced cases may require intravenous or subcutaneous fluid and electrolyte replacement at the veterinary clinic.

Other experts recommend feeding a home-prepared diet consisting of moderate amounts (50% or less) of high-quality, biologically appropriate protein. This includes fish, eggs, chicken, beef, or lamb. If possible, you may wish to alternate meals of mostly protein, with meals that are mostly vegetables. This allows the kidneys to rest during the low protein meals. In the case of a diabetic dog, it would be best to test blood glucose levels at home if you decide to use this method.

Treating Incontinence

There are several ways you can reduce the nuisance and number of urinary accidents around the house. Some methods involve behavior modification and dietary management. Others include physical aids and items that make living with chronic incontinence less troublesome.

Behavioral Issues and Incontinence

When you are home, pay attention to your dog's schedule, his water intake, and his body language. This is especially important for any dog suffering from polydipsia. Some dogs are better than others about "asking" to go out. They will make eye contact with you, wander near the door, or whine. Other dogs never ask. The owners of these dogs have to pay attention to the clock (when was the last time the dog went out?) and water consumption and encourage the dog to go again. Dogs typically need to urinate after activity (play), and often, after napping.

Have a specific word or phrase for elimination. There are times when it is helpful to have a dog eliminate upon command. Some owners say, "Do your business" or "Potty." You can help add this word to his vocabulary by saying, "good business" or "good potty," after he's done and by rewarding with a food treat. Keep treats handy.

If your dog does have an accident, do not carry on about it. Calmly help the dog out the door, and say whatever phrase you use for him to eliminate, reminding him that the outdoors is the appropriate place for this. In most cases, however, these are truly uncontrollable losses of urine and not lapses in house training.

Yelling or spanking can make a dog quite nervous about eliminating. A nervous dog is even less likely to ask to go out. You can clean up the accident while the dog is outdoors.

Cleaning Up Accidents

Deodorizing the spot reduces the chances of another accident happening in the same area. One of the oldest and best remedies is white vinegar. For urine accidents on carpet, repeatedly blot up the area. Lean your weight against small piles of towels, until no more appears to soak up.

Saturate the area with a mixture of 1/2 water and 1/2 vinegar, and cover it with a towel so that dirt is not tracked through the area. If the spot smells of anything other than the faint fragrance of vinegar after a day or two, repeat the process.

Dietary Issues and Incontinence

A number of dog owners report that dietary changes affect canine incontinence. They contend that eliminating grains from their dog's diet improved bladder control. This may be linked to the cycle of inflammation, cortisol production, and muscle weakness that grain protein is believed to induce.

Mechanical Aids and Items for Incontinence

If the accidents are frequent, consider making some concessions for your dog. If you do not have a doggy door to the yard, consider installing one, now. Consider purchasing housebreaking pads. These are a combination of absorbent paper toweling with a plastic backing. They are often scented so that puppies are attracted to eliminate on them. Similar pads are available in pharmacies or hospital supply stores for incontinent humans. These pads are larger in size than the puppy pads. If an older dog has repeated accidents in the same spot, you can put the pads there to protect that particular area in your house.

If there is a place in the house, garage, laundry room, etc., where you would be willing to let the dog relieve himself, put the pads there. Since most dogs do not like eliminating in the house once they have been housebroken, you may have to let your dog know that this spot is now acceptable to you.

Lead him to the spot at a time he normally eliminates, give him the command to eliminate...even if it is something such as, "Do you want to go out?" Tap the paper pads, and give him a food treat if he eliminates. You may even scent the pads with a few drops of his own urine if you collect it for other tests.

The owner of one large, geriatric dog was unable to make it home from work each day, before her dog needed to relieve himself. She set up a child's rigid, plastic swimming pool (the type that are about 8 to 10 inches high), lined it with newspapers, and placed it in her basement. Litter boxes designed specifically for dogs are available at some larger pet supply stores.

One owner, whose dog slept in another area of the house, purchased a baby monitor. With one monitor by the dog's bed, and one by hers, she was able to hear when the dog needed to go out at night.

Another owner purchased the type of rigid plastic carpet protector that fits underneath rolling desk chairs. In this way, she was able to hear the dog's toenails tap if the dog got out of bed during the night. The plastic served the dual purpose of preventing accidents in the dog's bed from leaking down onto the carpeting below. Plastic drop clothes and plastic-lined mattress pads can serve the same purpose. Mattress pads can also be used to cover favorite furniture.

Some people move the dog's sleeping quarters into a tiled or vinyl-floored bathroom. And there are certain dog beds available that will allow urine to pass through webbed bedding to a pan below. (See Supplier's section.)

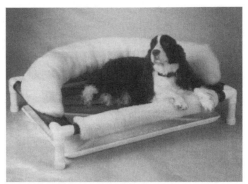

Some dog owners purchase or construct doggy diapers for incontinent pets. To diaper a male dog, purchase a regular diaper for human infants and several elastic dress clips, the type used to gather the fabric on the back of a dress. These are sold in fabric and fashion accessory stores.

Photo courtesy of SleePee-Time Beds

You can find similar elasticized clips designed to hold sheets on the bed in bed linen department. Apply the diaper like a cummerbund. You may line the diaper with feminine sanitary pads for additional absorbency. Diapers for female dogs are available commercially.

While some of these measures may seem extravagant, both dog and owner can benefit from them. Creating a situation where your dog can continue to be a clean and tidy pet improves the quality of his life, and probably yours as well.

Hepatic (Liver) Disease

The liver is involved in nearly all aspects of metabolism, so liver disease, regardless of cause, will affect almost every system in the body. The high levels of chemical additives found in commercial diets chronically irritate and strain the liver. This strain impairs the liver's ability to filter out debris and process food molecules in the bloodstream.

Once the body begins reacting to chronic inflammation (bowel, pancreas, and bladder), the liver must also filter out high levels of circulating hormones/steroids, such as adrenal estrogen and cortisol. Long-term cortisol (or prescription cortisone) can cause lesions to develop on the liver. The addition of any oral medications causes an even greater strain and workload.

Your veterinarian may recommend one of the many diagnostic measures to accurately diagnose your dog's liver problems. Blood work will evaluate blood cell counts and possible anemia. Blood chemistry analysis will examine the function of the liver as it attempts to process glucose, bilirubin, and urea. It will also evaluate electrolyte levels, albumin, globulin, and bile acid levels.

Measuring bile acids is considered one of the best tests available for evaluating liver function. Since little, if any, bile should escape the portal system (circulation between the liver, gallbladder, and intestine), any leakage is considered a sure sign of liver dysfunction. Other tests may include urine analysis, radiographs/x-rays, ultrasound, and liver biopsy.

Since the liver can regenerate itself, it is especially valuable to reduce the irritants that cause liver damage. Again consider switching to a homemade diet without grains, if you have not already done so. Liver lesions caused by high levels of cortisol *are* reversible, although it may take weeks, or even months.

Thyroid Disease

Hypothyroidism refers to the inability of the thyroid gland to produce sufficient thyroid hormone. The primary cause of hypothyroidism is lymphocytic thyroiditis, a condition in which white blood cells attack and destroy thyroid tissue. This is, perhaps, the most common autoimmune disease diagnosed in dogs today. Thyroid function is also affected (reduced) in the presence of excess cortisol or prescription cortisone. (See page 50.)

Like most other autoimmune diseases, there is likely a genetic component present in these cases, which is triggered by an environmental factor. Certain breeds seem more predisposed to thyroid disease. These include the Boxer, Doberman, English and Irish Setter, Clumber and Cocker Spaniel, Beagle, Poodle, Miniature Schnauzer, Labrador, Golden Retriever, Shetland Sheepdog (Sheltie), Old English Sheepdog, Chow Chow, and Akita. Of course, this list does not rule out the diagnosis of hypothyroidism in other breeds.

Signs of the disease include lethargy, weight gain, dry and brittle coat with increased shedding, cold intolerance (heat-seeking behaviors), hyperpigmentation of the skin, and neurological changes such as aggressiveness and seizures. There are numerous tests available for evaluating thyroid function and these are continually being updated and improved. Recent recommendations include the following tests to diagnose thyroid disease: total T4 (tT4), free T4 by equilibrium dialysis (fT4ed: a very accurate testing method), thyroglobulin autoantibodies (TgAA), and canine thyroid stimulating hormone (cTSH).

If your veterinarian diagnoses hypothyroidism, he will prescribe thyroid hormone supplements. Your dog will require one pill daily, as a life-long therapy. As with most other endocrine disorders, hypothyroidism is a condition that is *treated*, not cured.

Dogs that are diagnosed with both diabetes and hypothyroidism deserve some special consideration. Initiating thyroid treatment (supplementation) improves metabolism and frequently reduces the need for insulin. Diabetic dogs are typically started on lower than average levels of thyroid supplements. In addition, dosage requirements can change over the years and periodic re-testing is a good idea.

Calcinosis Cutis

Giving the appearance of a skin infection is the condition known as calcinosis cutis. This occurs in cases of hyperadrenocorticism when calcium is deposited in soft tissue and skin. Initially it may present as a white or cream-colored deposit. As it progresses, it may give the appearance of an allergic reaction and cause the dog extreme itching. These deposits are frequently located on the abdomen, base of the tale, and top of the neck.

The common reaction is to place the dog on steroid medication. This, however, just worsens the vicious cycle of rising cortisol levels. As Cushing's disease is brought under control, signs of calcinosis cutis should fade. Your veterinarian may also prescribe soothing shampoos and antihistamines to control the itching.

Ophthalmic Issues

It is interesting to note that a great number of autoimmune diseases have an impact on ocular health. It is crucial to consult a veterinarian who specializes in ophthalmology at the onset of eye problems. In fact, some dog owners access a specialist merely at the diagnosis of diabetes or Cushing's disease.

Board-certified veterinary ophthalmologists are specifically trained to diagnosis and treat ophthalmic disease. They receive a minimum of four years of specialty education. This greatly differs from the few weeks of ophthalmic study that is provided in general veterinary training.

Delaying ophthalmic care can have regrettable results. Many ophthalmic diseases are not self-limiting. If left untreated, they can lead to painful, expensive, and blinding conditions. If your veterinarian seems reticent to refer your dog to an ophthalmologist, you can certainly make such an appointment by yourself. Consult the phonebook, veterinary teaching hospital, or state veterinary association for a specialist.

Dietary therapy (supplementing with vitamins and minerals) is controversial subject. While it has not been proven to prevent or cure vision loss, some laboratory research suggests otherwise. Specifically, this refers to the addition of such minerals as zinc, and vitamins E. A, and C to the diet.

Ocular Anatomy

To discuss ophthalmic disease, a review of ocular anatomy is necessary. An understanding of the following terms will be helpful:

anterior chamber — the area between the cornea and the lens; and it is filled with a fluid called aqueous humor

aqueous humor — the fluid produced in the anterior chamber that maintains the shape of the chamber and nourishes the cornea

cataracts — changes in the lens fibers that result in opacity and blindness

choroid — made up mainly of blood vessels, one of the deep structural layers lining the back of the canine eye

ciliary body — the ocular structure that produces aqueous humor; it is located just posterior to the iris

cornea — the transparent structure at the very front of the eye, which allows light to pass further into the globe

filtration angle/trabecular meshwork — the structures in the eye that act as a drainage field through which aqueous humor escapes

iris — the structure that acts as an aperture, constricting and dilating in size in response to the amount of light present

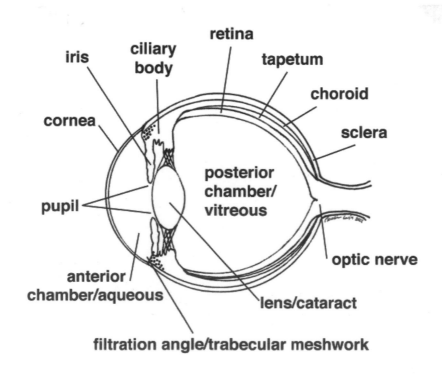

lens — the structure in the eye that helps to bend or refract rays of light and focus them upon the retina

lens capsule — a thin, transparent tissue that surrounds the lens

pupil — the area that appears as a black dot upon examination, but is actually the opening in the iris through which the posterior chamber may be viewed

retina — the inner-most structural layer of nerve cells (rods and cones) that lines the back of the eye and sends visual information to the brain

tapetum — another of the structural layers lining the back of the canine eye that reflects and amplifies light

vitreous humor — the gelatinous material that fills the posterior chamber of the eye

uvea (or uveal tract) — is made up of the iris, ciliary body, and choroid

Diabetic Cataracts

Cataracts are sometimes mistakenly described as a "film over the eye." This is not an accurate description. Dogs that develop cataracts experience a change in their lens tissue. The normally clear crystalline lens turns progressively white until it is completely opaque and obstructs the passage of light further into the eye. This white opacity is what we know as a cataract. If light can not reach the retina, the nerve tissue lining the back of the eye, images can not be perceived by the brain.

Cataracts occur in dogs for several reasons. In some cases, they are due to a genetic fault; in other cases, they are a result of normal aging. Diabetic cataracts are different from both of these. Diabetic cataracts are a result of metabolic problems. Because the body has difficulty metabolizing glucose, excess sugar accumulates in the lens of the eye. As it accumulates, it draws water into the lens with it. The accumulation of water breaks down the fibers of the lens, resulting in opacity.

Initially, a white glare in the dog's eyes may be noticeable in certain lighting. Eventually, the glare will be visible all the time. The pupil may become increasingly dilated, as it attempts to supply more light to the retina. Finally, the lens will be completely opaque, causing total blindness.

The timeline for developing diabetic cataracts can vary. Most experts believe that the sooner and better a dog's glucose levels are controlled, the greater the chance of forestalling cataract development. However, the majority of diabetic dogs will experience some lenticular changes within a year or two. Dog owners have witnessed cataract formation take several months to just a few days.

It is common and normal for dog owners to experience a sense of loss when cataracts are diagnosed. This is especially true for owners who have attempted to keep glucose levels tightly controlled. Dogs are typically less affected, psychologically, than are their owners.

Typical signs of vision loss can include bumping into objects, an unwillingness to do familiar activities (such as jumping into the car, running down the stairs), inability to catch a tossed item, and a change in attitude. Some dogs adjust quite well to the loss of vision. Others do not. If no complicating factors are present, surgical removal is most often the recommended treatment.

The veterinary ophthalmologist can make a more accurate diagnosis by performing a test called an electroretinogram (ERG). Much like an electrocardiogram (EKG), the procedure that measures heart function, an ERG measures the function of the retina. This test is extremely valuable since retinal degeneration sometimes coincides with cataract formation, aging, and endocrine diseases. An ophthalmologist will typically advise against cataract surgery if there is little or no retinal function determined by the ERG. It would be useless to remove the cataracts and allow light back into the eye if the retina were unable to process those light waves.

Many veterinary ophthalmologists are able to perform this procedure in essentially the same manner as it is performed on humans. Prior to cataract surgery, your dog may have steroid eyedrops prescribed. Steroids, even in topical form, may affect the blood glucose levels in sensitive individuals. Some diabetic dogs may require a slow and steady increase in insulin to remain regulated. One dog owner reported that a 30% increase in insulin was needed over a three-week period. Home blood glucose testing is a vital measure in keeping a dog regulated in situations like this.

To perform the cataract extraction, the surgeon makes an incision near the edge of the cornea and most often inserts the tip of a small instrument called a phaco-emulsifier. This is a pencil-sized instrument with a tiny cutting tip. It pulverizes the lens with ultrasound waves and then flushes away the fragments. Frequently, the surgeon implants a plastic intraocular lens (IOL). Follow-up exams are an important part of a successful recovery.

There are a few instances when surgery is not recommended. The first exception is in the case of hypermature cataracts. These eyes may be severely inflamed and are not good surgical candidates. Another exception is in a case when the ERG demonstrates no retinal function. Dogs with brittle, uncontrolled blood glucose levels may also be considered poor candidates, as well as those with severe heart problems.

In the case of long-standing, hypermature cataracts, the lens capsule may rupture and leak protein fragments into the globe of the eye. This may cause several additional problems. The protein fragments may obstruct the filtration angle, resulting in a condition known as glaucoma. (See page 150.) Fragments may cause severe inflammation, a condition known as lens-induced uveitis. (See page 150.) These two possible complications are important reasons to visit with a veterinary ophthalmologist at the onset of diabetes.

Two of the most common questions about cataract surgery include the expense and the outcome. Surgical quotes vary from practice to practice and from one part of the country and world to another. In addition, some practices quote a package price that includes the procedure, medications, follow-up visits, etc. Other clinics quote just the price of the surgery alone. Be sure to compare like costs, if doing comparative shopping.

Very roughly, in the United States, cataract extraction in a single eye can cost between $1,500 and $1,800. Removal of bilateral cataracts can run between $2,100 and $2,500. Additional variables include lens implants and, of course, any individual complications your dog may experience. Most clinics accept credit cards. Some offer payment plans.

Outcome for uncomplicated cataract extraction is usually improved vision and, often, dramatically so. Most dogs experience significant improvement in vision from just a few hours to a few weeks. (It can take up to two weeks to for the brain to adapt to new visual stimulus.) If your dog has additional ocular problems such as post-operative glaucoma, uveitis, or retinal detachment, the outcome may not be as good. It is important to remember that each dog is an individual and will heal differently.

Other considerations include that your dog may be required to wear an Elizabethan protection collar for several days or weeks. You will also be instructed to keep your dog's activity to a minimum. Both of these measures are aimed at protecting the eye during the healing process.

You will also have a medication regime to follow, post-operatively. This will include a variety of drops and ointments to reduce inflammation, promote healing, and prevent infection. All of this may affect your decision to proceed with surgery. If cataract extraction is not pursued, it is likely that the veterinary ophthalmologist will prescribe anti-inflammatory drops to prevent lens-induced uveitis.

Uveitis

Uveitis is the inflammation of the iris, ciliary body, or choroid. It can be caused by several factors. As previously described, inflammation can be lens-induced, as protein leaks from hypermature cataracts into the globe of the eye. Inflammation occurs because the body reacts to the lens protein as if it were a foreign invader. Uveitis can also occur in reaction to other systemic inflammation (autoimmune disease) or infection.

Signs of uveitis include redness of the "whites of the eyes" (the conjunctiva), watery eyes, squinting, blinking, low intra-ocular pressure, and rubbing of the face on paws or the carpet. Pain can be expressed as depression or loss of appetite. Treatment usually requires steroid treatment, either with oral medication or eyedrops. And as with other inflammatory conditions, uveitis can contribute to difficulty keeping diabetic dogs regulated.

Glaucoma

Glaucoma is a condition of fluid build up and abnormally high pressures within the eye. This usually occurs when the filtration angle (drainage field) no longer functions effectively.

If not treated quickly and correctly, increasing pressure can pinch off the blood vessels that nourish the retina and damage the optic nerve. As a result, the retinal cells eventually die and blindness results. Signs of glaucoma can include redness, cloudiness, bulging, dilated pupils, and loss of vision. The dog may squint or rub his eye(s) in an attempt to relieve pain.

Glaucoma is considered an emergency situation. If it is treated in time and correctly, vision can usually be maintained for some time. Treatment may initially include a wide variety of eye drops and oral medications to reduce the pressure and detect whether the eye has any remaining vision. Based on the findings, the veterinary ophthalmologist may recommend one of several surgical procedures for your dog. He may attempt to reduce the production of aqueous fluid by cryotherapy (freezing), laser treatment, or injection. These procedures scar or destroy the ciliary body and reduce aqueous production. Canine glaucoma is poorly controlled by medication, alone.

Sudden Acquired Retinal Degeneration (SARD)

SARD involves an abrupt loss of vision and the deterioration of retinal cells in both eyes. As the name implies, the onset of blindness is *quite* sudden. Owners report that their dogs seem to go blind overnight.

Upon visual inspection by the veterinary ophthalmologist, the dog's retinas appear normal at the onset of blindness. They can maintain this appearance until three to four months afterwards. At that time, the retinal cells often thin out until the greenish glow of the tapetum becomes visible. Following the initial, sudden onset of blindness, the disease does not progress significantly.

Typical behavioral signs of vision loss include bumping into objects, an unwillingness to do familiar activities (such as jumping into the car, running down the stairs), inability to catch a tossed item, and a change in attitude. Since there is usually no warning before the onset of SARD, there is little time for a dog to become accustomed to this change. Admittedly, sudden onset can cause a difficult adjustment to blindness. Aggressive and depressive behaviors are common.

SARD typically affects middle-aged animals, often in the range of 8 to 10 years. This disease usually results in complete and total blindness. While SARD can be emotionally and psychologically challenging for the dog, it is not a physically painful condition.

The cause of SARD is unknown, although it is assumed to be non-genetic. There exists some speculation in the veterinary community as to the connection between Cushing's disease and SARD. Signs suggestive of hyperadrenocorticism or Cushing's disease are often present. These include polydypsia (increased thirst), polyuria (excessive urination), polyphagia (increased hunger) weight gain, lethargy, and insomnia.

When laboratory blood tests are performed on SARD patients, the results can vary. Frequently, the results are normal. At other times lab tests can be negative for Cushing's disease initially, only to confirm Cushing's at a later time. In other instances, mild Cushing's signs are present at the onset of SARD, but later resolve themselves. In these cases, periodic retesting for Cushing's disease is recommended.

This author submits that SARD is part of the "threefold effect" caused by commercial pet food. (See page 54.) As with dry eye syndrome and diabetes mellitus, SARD *may* be an immune-mediated condition. But more likely, SARD is related to high levels of cortisol, combined with inadequate nutrition. Specifically, this would include the inability of some dogs to metabolize fat and fat-soluble vitamins, such as A and E, as well as various minerals. (See page 52.)

In humans, a gene called the p53 gene has been identified for it's role in destroying damaged or mutated cells in the body. It does this by initiating a "self-destruct" message, or **apoptosis**, inside the damaged cell. This process normally prevents the growth of cancer.

Cellular damage occurs for a variety of reasons, including chemical exposure, radiation exposure and inadequate nutrition. When the body detects such damage to a cell, cortisol crosses the cell membrane and initiates the programmed, self-destruct message. If this process is similiar in the canine body, then high levels of cortisol may be entering cells of the retina, damaged by inadequate nutrition, and programming them to self destruct.

The veterinary ophthalmologist may recommend that an electroretinogram (ERG) be performed. Much like an electrocardiogram (EKG) the procedure that measures heart function, an ERG measures the function of the retina. This test will help the doctor discern if the problem is with the retina (confirming the diagnosis of SARD), or if the problem involves the optic nerve or the brain.

There are recommended treatments for optic nerve inflammation and for brain cancer. At this time, there is no cure for SARD. A training program for blind dogs is the best form of treatment for dogs diagnosed with this condition. (See page 180.)

Dry Eye Syndrome (keratoconjunctivitis sicca or KCS)

This syndrome often occurs in Cushinoid and sub-Cushinoid dogs. As the name implies, dry eye syndrome results in reduced tear production, dryness, itchiness, and corneal ulcers. Another common sign of KCS is what dog owners term "goopy eyes," or the presence of green or light brown-colored mucous discharge. KCS is frequently misdiagnosed as an eye infection, but antibiotic treatment does not resolve the problem.

Like diabetes mellitus, KCS is yet another condition considered to have an immune-mediated basis. Antibodies that have been previously programmed to attack a foreign amino acid chain recognize and attack that same chain elsewhere in the body. In the case of KCS, the body attacks the tear-producing tissues of the eye.

In addition to evaluating the aforementioned signs, your veterinarian can perform a simple, painless test to diagnose KCS. This is called the Schirmer tear test and simply involves tucking small paper test strips under the dog's lower lid for 60 seconds. These test strips absorb and measure tear production. If tear production is below normal, your veterinarian will prescribe one or more drops or ointments.

KCS is commonly treated with cyclosporin drops. Cyclosporin is a medication thought to reduce the immune-mediated reaction. Other medications your veterinarian may prescribe are Optimmune drops or ointment (a milder form of cyclosporin), KCS drops, a combination of antibiotics, mucomyst (an ingredient that breaks up mucous), and a lubricant. Other medications may include oral pilocarpine (which stimulates tear production), Natural Tears, or Lacrilube (lubricating drops and ointments that are available without a prescription).

Applying Eye Drops

It may be necessary to give your dog eye drops in a variety of situations — before and after cataract surgery, as a preventive measure in cases of inoperable cataracts, in cases of dry eye syndrome, glaucoma, and uveitis. As with other medication techniques presented in this book, it can be helpful to practice before attempting to actually medicate your dog.

If your dog is wearing an Elizabethan cone/collar that makes it difficult to medicate him, remove it during the procedure. Let your dog nibble on a food treat. While he nibbles, approach the dog from behind. Stand by his side or straddle his back if possible.

Massage and pet your dog's head and neck. With the eye drop bottle in your dominant hand, reach around to steady the dog's head between both hands, and tilt his muzzle slightly upward. Quickly pull down the lower lid and pretend to express a drop.

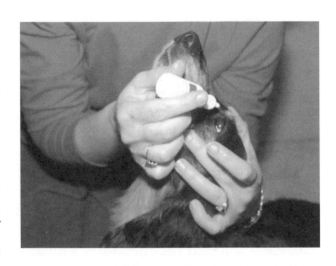

You may stop and offer him a food treat or continue on. Move your hands to the other side of his face and repeat. If yours is a highly active dog, move quickly. If you are straddling him, try to steady him between your legs.

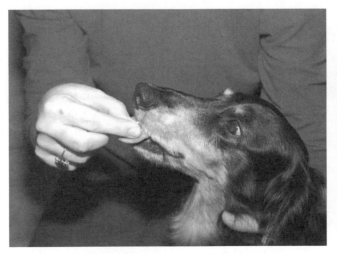
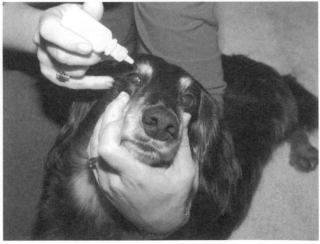

Reassuring comments may also prove helpful. Some dog owners keep a food treat close to the dog's face, either on a low table or chair, or have a family member hold it nearby. A final option, odd as it may sound, is to spread a small amount of peanut butter or cream cheese on the refrigerator door. This will distract the dog as well as help keep his head elevated.

Another method of applying eye drops involves having the dog lie down on his side. This places his eye on a very flat plane, and even if he blinks, the drop should fall onto the surface of the eye when he opens his lid. Of course, if both eyes require medication, you will need to position him twice, once on each side.

Surgical Considerations

Most veterinarians want a diabetic dog to be well regulated before any surgery is scheduled. Some believe that the surgical experience plays such havoc with blood glucose levels that it is acceptable to proceed with surgery, and regulate the diabetes afterward. The use of injectable anesthetics is typically avoided for diabetic dogs. Instead, inhalant anesthetics, such as Isoflourane gas are used.

Most often, dog owners are instructed to withhold food beginning at midnight the night before surgery. Consequently, your veterinarian will also have you withhold, or reduce by half, the morning dose of insulin.

Some veterinarians recommend that their clients slightly reduce insulin doses *after* the surgery, as an extra precaution. Other doctors recommend resuming the insulin schedule with the next meal. It is common for the stress and discomfort of surgery to elevate blood glucose levels. Avoid the temptation to increase insulin levels in response. With all of these influences, a dog can easily experience the Somogyi phenomenon after surgery.

Blood glucose levels are monitored during the surgical procedure as well as during recovery time. Glucose can be administered through intravenous fluids as needed. You should continue to monitor your dog carefully for several days after surgery. ✳

Closing

Emotional Support

Caring for a chronically ill pet is a labor of love. It can be emotionally exhausting. Not all of your friends, family, and co-workers will understand your commitment. Try to surround yourself with those who do.

Try to enjoy small pleasures with your dog and do not forget to take some time off for yourself and your own mental health. Enlist the help of others if you need a break from the role of caregiver. Burnout is a common side effect of providing long-term care.

A Word About Dog Training

Canine behaviors are best taught or modified by positive means, not punishment. If you are having difficulty dealing with your dog, first identify the problem behavior. Then using food treats, show the dog what you want him to do differently. Food and toys are powerful rewards for dogs.

If your dog views a situation as unpleasant or frightening, offer him food treats lavishly during that time. The dog will come to view the event as a rewarding experience. Be generous with your rewards. It is a good way to go through life.

Other Factors That Contribute to Canine Disease

In addition to a faulty, irritating diet and genetic predisposition, several other factors are believed to contribute to immune system failure. Environmental toxins and over-vaccination are two of these.

For years, the practice has been to inoculate pets on an annual basis. This repeatedly and unnecessarily provokes the immune response. Presently, veterinarians are departing from this philosophy. If you have an adult pet (older than 3 or 4 years of age), it is likely that he has developed lifelong immunity to the diseases for which he's been inoculated. Many veterinarians now recommend against vaccinating a dog that suffers from immune-related disease.

Environmental chemicals may also contribute to immune system dysfunction. It is common practice to use powerful pesticides on or near our pets. Some — such as flea bombs, carpet powders, weed killers, and garden pesticides — saturate the dog's environment. We place others directly on our pets: flea collars, shampoos, and repellents that are so potent they persist for many months. Keep in mind that the product labels instruct *humans* to wear gloves and wash their hands thoroughly after contact with these chemicals.

The canine body can adapt to years of biological stress, substituting one metabolic function for another. There are limits to everything, however. Sometimes it may seem as if serious illness is precipitated by a *single* stressor (e.g., vaccination, surgical procedure, insect bite). In reality, these events may just be the last straw, taxing a system that was ready to topple.

The Future

Every pet owner faces the day when his dog will be lost to illness, age or injury. It is a painful time for any animal lover. There are many good books devoted to the subject of pet loss, therefore, this topic will not be discussed at length here. However, the following story is offered in the hope that it provides the reader some small measure of comfort when that day arrives.

The Rainbow Bridge

There is a bridge connecting Heaven and Earth. It is called the Rainbow Bridge, because of its many colors. Just this side of the Rainbow Bridge, there is a land of meadows, hills, and valleys with lush green grass.

When a beloved pet dies, the pet goes to this place. There is always food and water and warm spring weather. The old and frail animals are young again. Those who are maimed are made whole again. They play all day with each other.

There is only one thing missing. They are not with their special person who loved them on Earth. So, each day they run and play until the day comes when one suddenly stops playing and looks up. The nose twitches. The ears are up. The eyes are staring. And this one suddenly runs from the group!

You have been seen, and when you and your special friend meet, you take him or her in your arms and embrace. Your face is kissed again and again and again, and you look once more into the eyes of your trusting pet. Then you cross the Rainbow Bridge together, never again to be separated.

Author Unknown

Some dog owners turn to new methods of animal husbandry after losing a pet to chronic illness. They embark on a more natural approach to dog feeding and health care. If you, too, are of this philosophy, seek out like-minded dog breeders. They can provide you with a puppy that has never been fed commercial food. This is important, since some of the most crucial damage appears to occur early in life. If you prefer mixed breeds, it is sometimes possible to adopt young puppies from animal shelters.

Whether your canine companions are puppies or adults, may your lives together be long. The human-canine bond is precious. None of us should lose a dog prematurely and none of our pets should needlessly suffer. ✻

Suppliers

American Eagle Food Machinery, Inc.
3557 South Halsted Street
Chicago, IL 60609-1606
Phone: (773) 376-0800
Toll free phone numbers:
    Order Hotline: (800) 836-5756,   Customer Service: (888) 390-0800
Web site: http://www.americaneaglemachine.com

Retailers of commercial-grade stainless steel meat grinders capable of grinding bones.

Aunt Jeni's Home Made Dog Food
PO Box 124
Temple Hills, MD 20757
Toll free: (877) 254-6123
Web site: http://www.auntjeni.com

In Canada:
Pets4Life
RR #4
Owen Sound, ONT N4K 5N6
Phone: (519) 372-1818
Web site: http://www.pets4life.com

Makers and distributors of *Home Made 4 Life* brand dog food, a prepared, frozen Bones And Raw Food diet.

Azmira Holistic Animal Care & Nutritional Products
2100 North Wilmot Road, Suite 109
Tucson, AZ 85712
Phone: (520) 886-8548
Toll free: (800) 497-5665
Web site: http://www.azmira.com

Holistic digestive aids: vitamin/mineral supplements, digestive enzymes, Panc'rse & Glucobalance drops, Stress & A'drenal Plex extract, Immuno Stim'r drops, and kidney/urinary tract formulas, canned and kibbled dog and cat food with human-grade meat.

B-Naturals
Natural and Holistic Supplements for Dogs and Cats
PO Box 217
Rockford, MN 55373
Phone: (763) 477-7001
Toll free (United States): (866) 368-2728
Web site: http://www.b-naturals.com

Braggs Organic Apple Cider Vinegar, PurePet Oatmeal Shampoo, Skin and Liver Plex, Kidni-Biotic, Kidni-Care, Cranberry Extract, Immune System Formula, HAC Immuno Stim'r, HAC Yeast and Fungal, HAC Blood & Lymph, HAC Stress & Adrenal, Berte's Immune Blend, Probiotics: Berte's Di-Acid Dim and Berte's Ultra Probiotic Powder.

Brandt P.P. Pants
715 Brandywine Drive
Lodi, CA 95240
Phone: (209) 368-6810
Web site: http://www.lodinet.com/pppants

Diapers for male dogs.

C & D Pet Products
405 East D Street
Petaluma, CA 94952
Phone: (707) 763-1654
Toll free: (888) 554-7387
Web site: http://www.cdpets.com

Carpeted pet steps, single or double, to help pets access furniture.

Commercial Matting/Consolidated Plastics Company, Inc.
8181 Darrow Road
Twinsburg, OH 44087
Toll free: (800) 362-1000

Mats and carpet runners with rubber backing.

Doctors Foster & Smith Inc.
2253 Air Park Road
Rhinelander, WI 54501-0100
Toll free: (800) 826-7206
Web site: http://www.drsfostersmith.com

Housebreaking pads, folding ramps for accessing trucks and RVs, dental care kits, Pet Pectate diarrhea control, urinary acidifier, pet bloomers and fancy pants (diapers for females), raised water and food bowls.

Holistic Pet Center
The Health Food Store for Pets
Box 1166
15599 SE 82nd Drive
Clackamas, OR 97015
Phone: (503) 656-5342
Web site: http://www.holisticpetcenter.com

Distributors of Vetline Veterinary Vitamins, which include, among other things, amino acids and glandular extracts of the thymus, liver, kidney, and adrenal glands. (Not for use with raw meaty bone diets however, as it would result in excess calcium intake.)

I.Q. Industries Inc.
737 Park Avenue
New York, NY 10021
Toll free: (877) 364-5438
Web site: http://www.dogramp.com

Heavy-duty, one-piece dog ramps with carpeting.

Maverick Marketing Ventures, Inc.
12550 Wolff Street
Broomfield, CO 80020
Phone: (303) 410-9020
Toll free (United States): (888) 244-5569
Web site: http://www.chillow.com

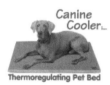

Canine Cooler Brand Thermoregulation Pet Bet – available in a variety of sizes and filled with water but due to their design, do not require refrigeration to keep pets cool.

Pinnacle Pet Supply
7251 PR 241 Mprtj
Cartier, MB R4K 1B4 Canada
Toll free (Canada): (877) 968-7738
Toll free (United States): (877) 668-7770
Web site: http://www.escape.ca/~pps/kooler.html

Kanine Kooler Pad — a 12" x 18" vinyl bag that is filled with water. It only weighs about 5 lbs., but it must be refrigerated to remain cool. The cooling effect is reported to last for approximately 2 hours.

Prozyme, Inc.
2567 Greenleaf Avenue
Elk Grove, IL 60007
Toll free: (800) 522-5537

Makers of digestive enzymes.

SleePee-Time Beds
2730 Willow Oak Circle
Charlottesville, VA 22901
Phone: (804) 296-1683
Toll free: (888) 824-7705
Web site: http://www.sleepeetime.com

Pet bed designed for incontinent animals.

Internet resources / discussion groups:

Blind dogs:
http://www.blinddogs.com

Cushinoid pets:
http://www.io.com/~loloawson/cushings/

Diabetic pets:
http://www.petdiabetes.org
http://http://www.mnsi.net/~queenie

Canine nutrition discussion group:
http://www.egroups.com/group.K9Nutrition

Glossary

acidophilus — a beneficial bacteria available as a dietary supplement

ACTH stimulation test — adrenocorticotrophic hormone stimulation test indicates the presence of hyperadrenocorticism

adipose – fatty body tissue

adrenal glands — two small endocrine glands located near the kidneys that secrete cortisol and adrenaline, as well as several other important hormones

adrenal tumor (AT) — the form of hyperadrenocorticism stemming from adrenal gland dysfunction

adrenalectomy — surgical removal of the adrenal glands

adrenocorticotrophic hormone (ACTH) — produced by the pituitary gland and primarily responsible for controlling cortisol secretion

amino acids — the building blocks of protein

amylase — enzyme (produced by the pancreas) responsible for digesting carbohydrates

apoptosis — programmed cell death

atrophy — withering of tissues and organs

autoimmune diseases (or immune-mediated condition) — the immune system's over-reaction to invaders, resulting in the destruction of the body's own cells and tissues

beta cells (or islet cells) — produce insulin in the endocrine pancreas

bile — a salty, yellowish fluid produced by the liver, stored in the gall bladder, necessary for the digestion of dietary lipids

bilirubin — a bile pigment derived from the breakdown of hemoglobin

bio-availability — a measure of how well nutrients are used by the body

biologically inactive hormone — a hormone that is unable to produce its expected effect in the body

calcinosis cutis — a condition, often accompanying Cushing's disease, in which calcium is deposited into the skin

catabolism — the effect cortisol has in breaking down muscle tissue to supply the body with glucose

cortisol — a natural steroid / hormone produced by the adrenal glands that is primarily responsible for ensuring the presence of glucose in the bloodstream

Cushing's disease — the pituitary-dependent form of hyperadrenocorticism (HAC) first identified by Dr. Harvey Cushing

diabetes insipidus — a disorder of water imbalance

digestive enzymes — natural chemicals produced by the body to break down food items into useable nutrients

dry eye syndrome — an autoimmune disease in which the body does not produce adequate or effective tear solution

electrolytes – substances such as sodium, potassium, chloride, and bicarbonate, which are found in blood and maintain the pH balance in the body

endocrine pancreas — the portion of the pancreas that produces insulin

endogenous ACTH test — a baseline measurement of the body's ACTH production

exocrine pancreas — the portion of the pancreas that produces digestive enzymes

false positive — a test result in which the patient falsely tests positive due to complicating factors or limitations of the test

fatty acids — the building blocks of dietary lipids

food enzymes — natural chemicals present in all fresh food that contribute to fermentation

food spike — a rise in blood glucose levels following a meal

glucagon — a hormone secreted by the pancreas that stores excess glucose in the liver and various large muscles

glucosuria — the presence of glucose in the urine

glycogen — the stored form of glucose

high dose dexamethasone suppression (HDDS) test — distinguishes between cases of adrenal-dependent and pituitary-dependent HAC

hyperadrenocorticism (HAC) — excess production of cortisol; also called Cushing's disease

hyperglycemia — high levels of blood glucose

hypertrophy — enlargement of tissues or organs from excessive use

hypoglycemia — low levels of blood glucose

hypothyroidism — insufficient thyroid function

iatrogenic — that which occurs as a side-effect of medication, not occurring naturally

immune-mediated conditions (or autoimmune diseases) — conditions stemming from the immune system's over-reaction to invaders

immunoglobulins — an important family of antibodies

immunoglobulin A (IgA) — considered to be the body's first line of defense and found in tears, saliva, and mucous membranes such as the lungs, urinary bladder, and the intestines

inflammatory bowel syndrome — a general term used to indicate chronic inflammation of the digestive tract

insulin dependent diabetes mellitus (IDDM) — the type of diabetes that can only be controlled by the injection of insulin, common in dogs

ketoacidosis — the metabolic state (highly acidic) caused by excess ketones present in the bloodstream

ketones (or **ketone acids**) — a by-product formed during the metabolism of body fat to glucose

ketonuria — the presence of ketones in the urine

leaky gut syndrome — the condition in which large protein molecules infiltrate the GI tract and initiate an autoimmune response

lipase — enzyme (produced by the pancreas) responsible for digesting fats (lipids)

lipolysis — the effect cortisol has in breaking down body fat to supply the body with glucose

low dose dexamethasone suppression (LDDS) test — distinguishes between cases of adrenal-dependent and pituitary-dependent HAC

lymphocytic thyroiditis — an autoimmune disease in which the immune system attacks the thyroid gland; a cause of hypothyroidism

melatonin — a natural hormone produced in the pineal gland responsible for wake/sleep cycles

metabolism / metabolic — the process by which food is chemically broken down and converted to energy for cell life

metabolic enzymes — natural chemicals present in the blood, tissues, and organs of the body that assist other chemical processes

mg/dL — milligrams per deciliter

non-insulin dependent diabetes mellitus (NIDDM) — the type of diabetes that can be controlled without the injection of insulin; rare in dogs

pancreatic enzyme test — measures levels of lipase, amylase, and pancreatic function

pancreatic exocrine insufficiency (PEI) (also called exocrine pancreatic insufficiency) — the inability of the exocrine pancreas to produce sufficient amounts of digestive enzymes

pancreatitis — the inflammation of the endocrine portion of the pancreas, either chronic or acute in nature

pituitary dependent — the form of hyperadrenocorticism stemming from pituitary gland dysfunction

polydipsia (PD) — excessive thirst

polyphagia (PP) — excessive hunger

polyuria (PU) — excessive urination

protease — enzyme (produced by the pancreas) responsible for digesting dietary proteins

renal threshold — the point at which the kidneys can no longer process glucose and it spills into the urine

resting cortisol level — the level of circulating cortisol read prior to tests for Cushing's disease

serum — the fluid of the blood

serum biochemical panel — measures liver enzymes and function

serum cholesterol and tryglyceride concentration test — indicates levels of lipids in the bloodstream

sudden aquired retinal degeneration (SARD) — sudden blindness frequently associated with Cushinoid symptoms

thyroid hormone — a natural hormone responsible for regulating the body's metabolic rate

total parenteral nutrition (TPN) — liquid nutrition supplied to the stomach via a feeding tube

trypsinogen-like immunoreactivity (TLI) **test** — measures trypsin and trypsinogen, two enzymes in the protease family, helpful in diagnosing cases of acute pancreatitis and pancreatic enzyme insufficiency

Type 1 diabetes mellitus — the type of diabetes caused by a destruction of pancreatic beta cells, usually requires insulin

Type 2 diabetes mellitus — the type of diabetes caused by either *defective* insulin molecules or by insulin resistance, *may* require insulin

urine cortisol creatinine ratio test — indicates Cushing's disease

Bibliography

Animal Protection Institute of America, "Pet Food Investigative Report," www.api4animals.org/petfood.htm, May 1996.

Billinghurst, Dr. Ian, BVSc (Hons), BscAgr., Dip. Ed., *Give Your Dog a Bone: The Practical Commonsense Way to Feed Dogs For a Long Healthy Life,* Australia, self-published, 1993.

Canine Health Foundation of the American Kennel Club, University of California at Davis, "International Symposium on Canine Hypothyroidism Report," www.goldens.com/tip8.html, August 3 & 4, 1996.

Feldman, Edward C., DVM, and Nelson, Richard W., DVM, *Canine and Feline Endocrinology and Reproduction, Second Edition*, Philadelphia, W.B. Saunders Company, 1996.

Goldstein, Martin, DVM, *The Nature of Animal Healing: The Path to Your Pet's Health, Happiness and Longevity*, New York, Alfred A Knopf, 1999.

Jackson, Gordon, MD, and Whitfield, Philip, MD, *Digestion: Fueling the System*, New York, Torstar Books, 1987.

Levin, Caroline D., RN, *Living With Blind Dogs: A Resource Book and Training Guide for the Owners of Blind and Low-Vision Dogs*, Oregon City, Lantern Publications, 1998.

Martin, Ann N., *Foods Pets Die For: Shocking Facts About Pet Food*, Troutdale, Oregon, New Sage Press, 1997.

Nelson, Richard W., DVM, Dip. ACVIM, and Couto, C. Guillermo, DVM, Dip. ACVIM, *Essentials of Small Animal Internal Medicine*, St. Louis, Mosby-Year Book, Inc., 1992.

Oldstone, Michael, BA, "Molecular Mimicry and Autoimmune Disease," *Cell*, 1987, vol. 50, pp. 819-820.

Olsen, Lew LMSW-ACP, PhD Natural Health, "Anatomy of a Carnivore and Dietary Needs," *B-Natural's Newsletter*, Spring 1999.

Palazzolo, Carl, DVM, "Cushing's Disease, (hyperadrenocorticism)," http://lbah.com/Canine/cushings.htm, September 20, 2000.

Plechner, Alfred J., DVM, *Pet Allergies: Remedies for an Epidemic*, Inglewood, Very Healthy Enterprises, 1986.

Richards, Michael, DVM, "Pancreatitis," www.vetinfo.com, June 9, 2000.

Santillo, Humbart, MH, ND, *Food Enzymes: The Missing Link to Radiant Health*, Prescott, Hohm Press, 1993.

Schultz, Kymythy R., AHI, *The Ultimate Diet: Natural Nutrition for Dogs and Cats*, Descanso, California, Affenbar Ink, 1998.

Scott, Fraser W., MD, et al., "Evidence for a Critical Role of Diet in the Development of Insulin-Dependent Diabetes Mellitus," *Diabetes Research*, 1998, vol. 7, pp. 153-157.

Strombeck, Donald R., DVM, PhD, *Home Prepared Dog & Cat Diets: The Healthful Alternative*, Ames, Iowa State University Press, 1999.

Volhard, Wendy, and Brown, Kerry, DVM, *The Holistic Guide for a Healthy Dog*, New York, Howell Book House, 1995.

Zaahradnik, Robert T., PhD, "Calcium and Magnesium: Important Macrominerals," www.vitality.simplenet.com/health/drzaah.htm, December 23, 2000.

Index

A

Accidents in the house
  Cleaning up 141
Acid / alkaline relationship 34
Acidify agents 139
ACTH 12, 49
  Feedback loop 49
ACTH Stimulation Test 28, 125
Adrenal gland 12, 23
Adrenal tumors 26, 30
Adrenocorticotrophic hormone. *See* ACTH
Aggression. *See* Mood changes
Alkaline phosphatase 21
Allergic reactions 49
Amino acids 15, 48, 51
  Altered 44
Amylase. *See* Enzymes
Anatomy 11
Apoptosis 151
Appetite center 36
Auto-digestion 33
Autoimmune disease 20, 51
Autoimmune hemolytic anemia 51

B

Bacteria 41, 139
Bacteriuria 21
Behavioral changes. *See* Mood changes
Beta cells 14, 20, 51
BHA 46
BHT 46
Bile 12, 16, 21, 34, 51. *See also* Vomiting: Of bile
Bilirubin 12, 21, 143
Bioavailability 45
Biologically appropriate 46
Bladder infections *See* Urinary tract infections
    (UTIs)
Blindness 25. *See also* Ophthalmic issues
Blood chemistry analysis 143
Blood clots 49
Blood glucose. *See* Glucose
Body weight
  Changes in 70, 144

C

Calcinosis cutis 25, 145
Calcium 13, 25, 140
  Deposits 49
  Stones 25
  Supplements 60
Carbohydrates 14, 23, 46
Catabolism 14, 24
Cataracts 18, 147
Cholesterol 59
Circadian rhythm 25
Circling behavior 25
Coat
  Changes in 25, 144
Colitis 36
Colon 12
Combination dexamethasone suppression and ACTH
    stimulation test 30
Confusion. *See* Mood changes
Cooling pads 127
Cortisol 12, 14, 23, 49
  Biologically inactive 49, 50
  Circadian rhythm 25
  Continuum 53
Cortisone 23
Cushing's disease 23, 151
Cushing's tests 30, 49
  ACTH stimulation test 28
  False readings 49, 50
  Low dose dexamethasone suppression (LDDS)
    test 29
  Urinary cortisol creatinine ratio test (UCCR) 30
Cyclosporin 152

D

Demineralization 25, 140
Dental health 24
  Gingivitis 137
  Gums 24, 138
Depression. *See* Mood changes
Dexamethasone 29
Diabetes insipidus 19

Diabetes mellitus 17
  Causes 19
  Diagnosing 21
  Types of diabetes 19
    Insulin dependent 19
    Non-insulin dependent 19
    Type 1 19
    Type 2 19
Diarrhea 34, 36, 52
  Control of 59
Diets 39
  Commercial 39
    Chemicals 46
    "Consumer Digest" report 55
    Fats in 51
    Fiber in 45
    Grains in 46
    Guidelines for owners 55
    Meat by-products in 42
    Protein sources in 42
  Holistic 39
  Home-cooked 57
    For dogs With Kidney Disease or Pancreatitis 58, 140
    Reduced need for insulin 61
  Homemade
    Transition to 71
    Variations in 66
  Premium 39, 47
  Prescription 39, 47
  Raw 62
    Bacteria 63
    Feeding bones 62
    Insulin reduction 65
  Switching 66
Digestive enzymes. *See* Enzymes
Digestive system 40
  Slowed digestion 44
Disseminated intravascular coagulation 35
DNA 41
Doctor-client relationship 7
  The dog owner's part 8
  The veterinarian's part 7
  Treatment philosophies 8
Dog food. *See* Diets: Commercial
Dog training 92, 155
Dry eye syndrome 18, 25, 152

E

Ear infections 137
Electrolyte imbalance. *See* Ketoacidosis
Electroretinogram (ERG) 151
Emotional support 155
Endogenous ACTH test 31

Enzymes 21, 42, 43
  Activate 14, 33
  Digestive
    Amylase 12, 13, 21, 47
    Lipase 12, 13, 21
    Protease 12, 13, 15
  Elevated levels 37
  Food/ intrinsic 43, 66
  Metabolic 21, 42
    Liver 21, 35
Epileptic seizures 25, 144
Estrogen 50
  Adrenal 50
Ethoxyquin 46
Excess hunger. See Polyphagia
Exercise and the diabetic 120
Eye problems. See Ophthalmic issues

F

Fats 15
Fats (Lipids) 15, 33, 51
Finicky eaters 56
Fructosamine test 119

G

Gallbladder 12, 15
Gastrointestinal (GI) tract 11
Glaucoma 150
Glucose 14
  Blood glucose 14
    Hyperglycemia 18. See also Hyperglycemia
    Hypoglycemia 98, 118
    Milligrams per deciliter 15
    Millimoles per liter 15
    Normal range 14
    Regulating 100, 102, 115, 117, 139, 154
Glucose testing 103
  At the veterinary clinic 101
  Home blood 105
    Evaluating a curve 113
    Helpful hints 111
    How to perform 108
    Lancets 106
    Meters 107
    When to do a curve 113
    When to do spot checks 112
  Urine 103
Glucosuria 18, 21
Glycogen 14
Glycosylated hemoglobin test. 119
Grain 46, 48, 141
  Oatmeal 59
Grief. *See* loss
Grinders. *See* Meat grinding machine

H

Hearing impairment 25
Heart 24
    Arrhythmia 35
    Failure 24
Heat intolerance 24
High dose dexamethasone suppression (HDDS) test
    30
High-cortisol continuum 151. *See also* Cortisol
Histamine 48
Honeymoon period 116
Hyperadrenocorticism 27. *See also* Cushing's
    disease
    Comfort measures 127
    Diagnosing 27
        ACTH stimulation test 28
        Combination dexamethasone suppression and
        ACTH stimulation test 30
        Endogenous ACTH test 31
        High dose dexamethasone suppression (HDDS)
        test 30
        Low dose dexamethasone suppression (LDDS)
        test 29
        Urinary cortisol creatinine ratio test 30
    Treatment 123
    Types of Hyperadrenocorticism
        Adrenal-dependent 26
        Iatrogenic hyperadrenocorticism 26
        Pituitary-dependent 26, 30
    Types of Hyperadrenocorticism
    Types of Hyperadreno 26
Hyperglycemia 18
Hyperparathyroidism 25
Hypoglycemia 98, 117
Hypothyroidism 18. *See also* Thyroid: Disease

I

IgA. *See* Immunoglobulins
IgA deficiency 48, 50, 138
IgE. *See* Immunoglobulins
IgG. *See* Immunoglobulins
IgM. *See* Immunoglobulins
Immune system 20
    Immune-system function 11, 24, 47, 49, 50, 156
Immune-mediated conditions 20
Immunoglobulins 47
    Immunoglobulin A (or IgA) 48
    Immunoglobulin E (or IgE) 48
    Immunoglobulin G (or IgG) 48
    Immunoglobulin M (or IgM) 48
Incontinence. *See* Urinary incontinence
Increased appetite. *See* Polyphagia
Increased thirst. *See* Polydipsia

Increased urination. *See* Polyuria
Infections 43, 49
    Dietary management of 139
    Ear 137
    Kidney 140
    Oral 137
    Skin 137
    Urinary tract (UTIs) 49, 138
Inflammatory bowel disease 34, 36, 49, 66
Insulin 14, 23
    Activity 73
        Duration 74
        Intermediate-acting 75
        Long-acting 75
        Nadir 74
        Onset 74
        Peak 74
        Short-acting 74
    Animal-based 76
    Bottles and labels 80
    Changing types of 115
    Human-based 77
    Injections 77
        Changing doses 104, 114
        Gone wrong 96
        How to prepare 84
        Procedure description 89
        Rotating injection sites 88
        Timing meals with 77
        Training the dog 92
    Resistance 24, 116
    Schedule flexibility 79
    Storage and handling 83
    Syringes
        Pre-filling 87
    Syringes and needles 81
Intestinal wall
    Permiability 48
Islet cells. *See* Beta cells

J

Jaundice 35

K

Ketaconazole 126
Ketoacidosis 17, 119
Ketones 17
Ketonuria 17, 21
Kidney 12
    Degeneration 45, 66, 140
        Cause 45, 140
    Failure 35
Kidney infection 140

L

L-Deprenyl. *See* Anipryl
Laboratory tests 21
  Complete blood count 21
  Pancreatic enzyme tests 21
  Serum biochemical panel 21
  Serum cholesterol and triglyceride concentration 21
  Urinalysis 21
Lameness 140
Large intestine 12, 52
Leaky gut syndrome 51, 53
Lecithin 59
Lipase. *See* Enzymes
Lipids. *See* Fats
Lipolysis 14, 24
Liver 12, 14, 33
  Disease 45, 49, 143
    Causes 143
    Diagnosing 143
    Treating 144
  Disseminated intravascular coagulation 35
  Enzymes 21
  Function 21, 66
  Lesions 25, 143
Loading phase. *See* Lysodren
Loss 1, 148
  Acceptance 3
  Anger 2
  Bargaining 3
  Denial 2
  Depression 3
Loss of appetite 56, 140, 150
Low dose dexamethasone suppression (LDDS) test 29
Lungs. *See* Pulmonary
Lymphatic system 13, 16, 33, 52
Lymphocytic thyroiditis 144
Lysodren 124
  Trouble with 130

M

Magnesium 13, 18, 24, 34, 50, 60, 140
Malabsorption 34, 36
Mats and carpet runners 129
Meals 115
  Changing mealtimes 115
  Timing insulin injections with 78
Meat by-products 42
Meat grinding machine 64
Medication 130
  Anipryl 126
  Cyclosporin 152
  Ketaconazole 126

Lysodren 124
Melatonin 25
Metabolic enzymes. *See* Enzymes
Metabolism 11, 13
  Abnormal 17, 23, 33
Mitotane. *See* Lysodren
Mood changes 25, 35, 144, 150, 151
Muscle weakness 128. *See also* Catabolism

O

Oatmeal 59
Ophthalmic issues 145
  Cataracts 147
  Dry eye syndrome (keratoconjunctivitis sicca or KCS) 152
  Electroretinogram (ERG) 151
  Eye drops
    How to apply 152
  Glaucoma 150
  Ocular anatomy (parts of the eye) 145
  Uveitis 150
Oral Infections 137
Oral supplements. *See* Supplements

P

Pancreas 11, 13
  Endocrine pancreas 12, 14
  Exocrine pancreas 12, 33
Pancreatic disease 33
  Cysts and abscesses 35
Pancreatic duct 14
Pancreatic exocrine insufficiency 35
Pancreatitis 35
  Causes of 36
  Diagnosing 37
  Types of 35
    Acute 35
    Chronic 35
Parathyroid gland 25
Pepsin 15
Phosphorus 13, 140
Physical assessment 135
Pineal gland 25
Pituitary gland 13, 23
Polydipsia 18, 24, 138
Polyphagia 17, 24
Polyuria 18, 24, 50, 138, 140
Portal system 15, 143
Potassium 24, 34
Protease. *See* Enzymes
Proteins 15, 45
Proteinuria 21
Pulmonary edema 49
Puppies 157

Intestinal wall 48, 51

R

Raised bowls 129
Ramps 128
Reading list 72
Receptors 14
Renal. *See* Kidney
Renal threshold 18
Ricinoleic acid 52

S

Seizures. *See* Epileptic seizures
Sharps disposal containers 83
Skin 137, 145
    Calcinosis cutis 25, 145
    Infections 137
    Thinning 25, 144
Small intestine 11, 13
Snacks and treats 67
Somogyi phenomenon 117. See also Glucose:
    Blood glucose: Regulating
Stomach 11
Stomach acid 41
Stupor 25. *See also* Mood changes
Sudden Acquired Retinal Degeneration (SARD) 150
Suggested reading materials 72
Supplements 60
    Acidifying 139
    Calcium and phosphorus 60, 65
    Glandular extracts 70
    Melatonin 71
    Phosphatidyl serine 71
Surgical procedures and the diabetic 154

T

Teeth (dentition). *See* Dental health
Threefold effect of commercial food 151
Thyroid 50
    Disease 144
        Hypothyroidism 51
        Lymphocytic thyroiditis 51, 144
    Hormone 50
    Inactive 50
Training the dog 95
    The down-stay 96
    The sit-stay 95
Traveling with a diabetic 121
Trypsinogen-like-immunoreactivity (or TLI) test 37
Tumors 50

U

Urea 143
Urinary cortisol creatinine ratio test 30

Urinary glucose 103
Urinary incontinence 24, 138, 140
    Cleaning up accidents 141
    Dietary issues 141
    Mechanical aids and items 142
Urinary tract infections (UTIs) 138
Urine pH 139
Urine sample 138
    How to collect 104, 138
Uveitis 25, 150

V

Vaccinations 155
Vegetables 60
    High in potassium 60
    High in sugar 60
    Pulping 59
Vitamin A 13, 52
Vitamin B 13
Vitamin C 13, 52
Vitamin D 13, 52
Vitamin E 13,52, 60, 145
Vomiting 34, 140
    Of bile 34, 51

W

Water consumption 69
    Monitoring average daily 103, 125
Weight
    changes in 36, 70
White blood cells 21, 35, 37, 43, 50
Wolf 40, 63
    Diet of 45, 48

Notes

O   10r

"Living With Blind Dogs: A Resource Book and Training Guide for the Owners of Blind and Low-Vision Dogs" by Caroline D. Levin

8.5"x 11" paperback, 182 pages, illustrated, ISBN 0-9672253-0-2

 This is the first-ever resource book of its kind. It embodies helpful hints from dozens of blind-dog owners, as well as years of ophthalmic nursing, veterinary, and dog training experiences. Topics include dealing with loss, causes of blindness, how dogs react to blindness, pack interactions, training new skills, toys and games, and more.

Price: $29.95 plus shipping & handling $5.95 (U.S. & Can.), $15.95 elsewhere

---

"Blind Dogs Stories: Tales of Triumph Humor and Heroism" by Caroline D. Levin

5.5"x 8.5" paperback, 100 pages, illustrated, ISBN 0-9672253-1-0

 Two dozen short stories, collected from around the world – some of them humorous, some of them heroic, all of them heartwarming. This book demonstrates that blind dogs can live useful and happy lives, offers encouragement to blind-dog owners, and celebrates the beauty of the human-canine bond.

Price: $12.95 plus shipping & handling $5.95 (U.S. & Can.), $15.95 elsewhere

---

Shipment is by Priority Mail: 1-3 day delivery in the U.S. For credit card orders, please phone, fax, or visit our website. Make checks payable, (in U. S. funds, on U.S. banks, please) and mail to:

Caroline Levin
Lantern Publications
18709 S. Grasle Road
Oregon City, OR 97045-8899 USA

phone and fax: (503) 631-3491
email: publisher@petcarebooks.com
website: http://www.petcarebooks.com